FAST FACTS FOR THE
CLINICAL NURSING INSTRUCTOR

Eden Zabat Kan, PhD, RN, received her bachelor's degree in nursing from Penn State University at State College, PA, her master's degree in nursing education from Villanova University, Villanova, PA, and her doctorate in nursing science from Widener University, Chester, PA. She is currently employed at the School of Nursing at the Catholic University of America in Washington, DC.

Susan Stabler-Haas, MSN, APRN-BC, is an adjunct faculty member at Villanova University. She is a Villanova graduate and has over 25 years of classroom and clinical teaching experience in the areas of medical-surgical, critical care, geriatric, and psychiatric nursing. Her instruction is influenced by her prior roles as staff nurse, rehabilitation nurse, and critical care nurse manager in five Philadelphia-area hospitals. She has educated students in a variety of nursing programs, including diploma, associate, baccalaureate, RN to BSN, and second degree nursing. Professor Stabler-Haas has earned a psychiatric clinical nurse specialist designation from the University of Pennsylvania. She is a licensed marriage and family therapist, incorporating mindfulness in her practice.

Fast Facts for the NEW NURSE PRACTITIONER: *What You Really Need to Know in a Nutshell, 2e* (Aktan)

Fast Facts for the ER NURSE: *Emergency Room Orientation in a Nutshell, 2e* (Buettner)

Fast Facts for the MEDICAL–SURGICAL NURSE: *Clinical Orientation in a Nutshell* (Ciocco)

Fast Facts for the NURSE PRECEPTOR: *Keys to Providing a Successful Preceptorship in a Nutshell* (Ciocco)

Fast Facts for the OPERATING ROOM NURSE: *An Orientation and Care Guide in a Nutshell* (Criscitelli)

Fast Facts for the ANTEPARTUM AND POSTPARTUM NURSE: *A Nursing Orientation and Care Guide in a Nutshell* (Davidson)

Fast Facts for the NEONATAL NURSE: *A Nursing Orientation and Care Guide in a Nutshell* (Davidson)

Fast Facts About PRESSURE ULCER CARE FOR NURSES: *How to Prevent, Detect, and Resolve Them in a Nutshell* (Dziedzic)

Fast Facts for the GERONTOLOGY NURSE: *A Nursing Care Guide in a Nutshell* (Eliopoulos)

Fast Facts for the LONG-TERM CARE NURSE: *What Nursing Home and Assisted Living Nurses Need to Know in a Nutshell* (Eliopoulos)

Fast Facts for the CLINICAL NURSE MANAGER: *Managing a Changing Workplace in a Nutshell* (Fry)

Fast Facts for EVIDENCE-BASED PRACTICE: *Implementing EBP in a Nutshell, 2e* (Godshall)

Fast Facts About NURSING AND THE LAW: *Law for Nurses in a Nutshell* (Grant, Ballard)

Fast Facts for the L&D NURSE: *Labor & Delivery Orientation in a Nutshell, 2e* (Groll)

Fast Facts for the RADIOLOGY NURSE: *An Orientation and Nursing Care Guide in a Nutshell* (Grossman)

Fast Facts on ADOLESCENT HEALTH FOR NURSING AND HEALTH PROFESSIONALS: *A Care Guide in a Nutshell* (Herrman)

Fast Facts for the FAITH COMMUNITY NURSE: *Implementing FCN/Parish Nursing in a Nutshell* (Hickman)

Fast Facts for the CARDIAC SURGERY NURSE: *Everything You Need to Know in a Nutshell* (Hodge)

Fast Facts for the CLINICAL NURSING INSTRUCTOR: *Clinical Teaching in a Nutshell, 2e* (Kan, Stabler-Haas)

Fast Facts for the WOUND CARE NURSE: *Practical Wound Management in a Nutshell* (Kifer)

Fast Facts About EKGs FOR NURSES: *The Rules of Identifying EKGs in a Nutshell* (Landrum)

Fast Facts for the CRITICAL CARE NURSE: *Critical Care Nursing in a Nutshell* (Landrum)

Fast Facts for the TRAVEL NURSE: *Travel Nursing in a Nutshell* (Landrum)

Fast Facts for the SCHOOL NURSE: *School Nursing in a Nutshell, 2e* (Loschiavo)

Fast Facts About CURRICULUM DEVELOPMENT IN NURSING: *How to Develop & Evaluate Educational Programs in a Nutshell* (McCoy, Anema)

Fast Facts for DEMENTIA CARE: *What Nurses Need to Know in a Nutshell* (Miller)

Fast Facts for HEALTH PROMOTION IN NURSING: *Promoting Wellness in a Nutshell* (Miller)

Fast Facts for STROKE CARE NURSING: *An Expert Guide in a Nutshell* (Morrison)

Fast Facts for the MEDICAL OFFICE NURSE: *What You Really Need to Know in a Nutshell* (Richmeier)

Fast Facts for the PEDIATRIC NURSE: *An Orientation Guide in a Nutshell* (Rupert, Young)

Fast Facts About the GYNECOLOGICAL EXAM FOR NURSE PRACTITIONERS: *Conducting the GYN Exam in a Nutshell* (Secor, Fantasia)

Fast Facts for the STUDENT NURSE: *Nursing Student Success in a Nutshell* (Stabler-Haas)

Fast Facts for CAREER SUCCESS IN NURSING: *Making the Most of Mentoring in a Nutshell* (Vance)

Fast Facts for the TRIAGE NURSE: *An Orientation and Care Guide in a Nutshell* (Visser, Montejano, Grossman)

Fast Facts for DEVELOPING A NURSING ACADEMIC PORTFOLIO: *What You Really Need to Know in a Nutshell* (Wittmann-Price)

Fast Facts for the CLASSROOM NURSING INSTRUCTOR: *Classroom Teaching in a Nutshell* (Yoder-Wise, Kowalski)

Forthcoming FAST FACTS Books

Fast Facts for TESTING AND EVALUATION IN NURSING: *Teaching Skills in a Nutshell* (Dusaj)

Fast Facts for the CLINICAL NURSE MANAGER: *Managing a Changing Workplace in a Nutshell, 2e* (Fry)

Fast Facts for the CARDIAC SURGERY NURSE: *Caring for Cardiac Surgery Patients in a Nutshell, 2e* (Hodge)

Fast Facts About the NURSING PROFESSION: *Historical Perspectives in a Nutshell* (Hunt)

Fast Facts for the HOSPICE NURSE: *A Concise Guide to End-of-Life Care* (Wright)

Visit www.springerpub.com to order.

FAST FACTS FOR THE CLINICAL NURSING INSTRUCTOR

Clinical Teaching in a Nutshell

Second Edition

Eden Zabat Kan, PhD, RN
Susan Stabler-Haas, MSN, APRN-BC

SPRINGER PUBLISHING COMPANY
NEW YORK

Springer Publishing Company, LLC
11 West 42nd Street
New York, NY 10036
www.springerpub.com

Acquisitions Editor: Margaret Zuccarini
Composition: S4Carlisle Publishing Services

ISBN: 978-0-8261-1894-3
E-book ISBN: 978-0-8261-1899-8

15 / 5 4

The author and the publisher of this Work have made every effort to use sources believed to be reliable to provide information that is accurate and compatible with the standards generally accepted at the time of publication. Because medical science is continually advancing, our knowledge base continues to expand. We recommend that the reader always consult current research and specific institutional policies before performing any clinical procedure. The author and publisher shall not be liable for any special, consequential, or exemplary damages resulting, in whole or in part, from the readers' use of, or reliance on, the information contained in this book. The publisher has no responsibility for the persistence or accuracy of URLs for external or third-party Internet websites referred to in this publication and does not guarantee that any content on such websites is, or will remain, accurate or appropriate.

Library of Congress Cataloging-in-Publication Data

Kan, Eden Zabat, author.
 Fast facts for the clinical nursing instructor : clinical teaching in a nutshell / Eden Zabat Kan, Susan Stabler-Haas. —Second edition.
  p. ; cm.
 Includes bibliographical references and index.
 ISBN-13: 978-0-8261-1894-3
 ISBN-10: 0-8261-1894-1
 ISBN-13: 978-0-8261-1899-8 (e-book)
 I. Stabler-Haas, Susan, author. II. Title.
  [DNLM: 1. Education, Nursing—methods. 2. Teaching—methods.   WY 18]
  RT71
 610.73071'1—dc23

2013008724

Printed in the United States of America by Gasch Printing.

Contents

Part VIII: The Growing Importance
of Reference Letters and Simulation

Foreword

Each of us has significant memories of our nursing school experience. Maybe we remember the clinical instructor who talked us through giving our first injection or insertion of a Foley catheter. Maybe we remember "shaking in our boots" for fear that we would be unprepared to answer our instructor's question with what we perceived to be a "stupid answer." It is hoped that in all of these cases, we remember the importance of quality nursing and how much we learned from the instructors who dedicated their lives to providing positive learning experiences in the clinical setting.

The education of nursing students requires a balance between theoretical knowledge and clinical application—what some refer to as the science and art of nursing. Many nursing faculty members perform both of these roles within the nursing program, but as financial constraints increase, many colleges and universities have hired adjunct faculty who work only in the clinical facility with nursing students. Many of these individuals have significant clinical expertise, but they may lack the knowledge and skill to convey that expertise to students. Some faculty have not completed the graduate courses that support the teaching role, such as courses in curriculum, tests and measurements, creative teaching strategies and, most importantly, the teaching practicum experience, in which graduate students are placed in colleges and universities for a semester to learn the role of the nursing faculty member.

We all have to start somewhere, and I suspect some of you can remember your first clinical teaching position. The best clinical instructors make the job look easy, and most people don't realize how much effort goes into the process of clinical teaching to create a positive learning environment for the nursing student. This book provides readers with a framework of ideas that will help them prepare for clinical teaching, including organizing the clinical experience, developing relationships with the staff in the clinical facilities, making clinical assignments, planning orientation days, developing clinical rotations, planning and facilitating pre- and postconferences, making clinical evaluations, discussing legal issues of clinical education and, of course, handling the student who is in jeopardy of failing the clinical course. The clinical instructor carries the additional burden of accountability—ensuring that each student is providing safe and effective nursing care to patients. As a result, issues of personal liability and techniques for handling the student who is in jeopardy of giving unsafe care become important. Picture yourself teaching 8 to 10 nursing students on a busy medical-surgical unit. If each student carries two to three patients, you quickly become aware of how challenging this responsibility can be. No wonder I have heard more than a few graduate students during their teaching practicum experience express surprise when they say, "I never knew how much work went into teaching!" I would be remiss if I didn't mention Teresa Christian as a shining example of these clinical nursing instructors. Many Villanova University alumni have described her as "tough, but the best instructor I ever had!"

The idea for this book began with discussions over coffee between two faculty members who had a similar philosophy about clinical instruction. They shared a commitment to making the clinical experience the best it could be for their students, making improvements every year they taught. In addition, they were often assigned the task of orienting and mentoring new clinical faculty. The authors agreed that what was missing in the literature was a "real-life" practical guide to assist new faculty in transitioning from clinical practice to clinical education. From those early discussions and a lot of brainstorming, this book became a reality.

This book serves as a valuable resource for nurses who are beginning their professional teaching careers and for seasoned faculty who seek additional resources to improve the clinical experience for their students. In many ways, this book is a tribute to the clinical aspects of our nursing programs and to the clinical faculty members who strive to make the student experience a positive one. This book was written by two of the best clinical faculty members I have ever known. I have learned much from them in my own practice, and I am confident that you will also grow from their combined experience and wisdom. There is no question that you will find in these pages a wealth of pragmatic, "real-life" information on the clinical teaching process.

I want to thank Eden Zabat Kan and Susan Stabler-Haas for asking me to write the Foreword for the second edition of this book. It is indeed an honor to be a small part of this significant contribution to the nursing education literature. The authors have made revisions to each original chapter, as well as added chapters on reference writing and clinical simulation experiences. I am confident this book will help you to become one of those clinical instructors that students will look back on with pride and say, "That clinical instructor made me the nurse I am today!"

Susan C. Slaninka, EdD, RN
Adjunct Professor of Nursing
Villanova University College of Nursing

Preface

Let's face it. Not every nurse would make a good clinical instructor. Technical proficiency alone does not guarantee the ability to effectively manage nursing students at the clinical site. Even nurses who are capable of providing clinical instruction may not wish to take on the considerable personal liability associated with the oversight of these nursing students.

Perhaps you are different. Perhaps you are a nurse who is both capable and willing to impart your knowledge to the next generation of caregivers. We commend you, for the future of our profession rests on your shoulders. After all, what is more important to the future of nursing than supervising and sharing our expertise with future nurses?

While personally rewarding, this vital role is also a formidable challenge. Clinical teaching is not easy. The expectations for an effective clinical nursing instructor are daunting. It can be a prodigious undertaking even for individuals with training or degrees in clinical instruction. They are continually faced with the changing demands of the patient and the challenges of adapting instruction to different learning styles. Moreover, most new clinical instructors do not have a solid foundation in teaching clinical courses. Indeed, many may not have any teaching experience. As a result, they face performance insecurities, along with the daily teaching challenges.

It is easy to understand why nursing programs are pressed to fill their clinical instructor positions.

Fast Facts for the Clinical Nursing Instructor: Clinical Teaching in a Nutshell, second edition, is designed as a practical guide for clinical instructors addressing key fundamental elements of clinical teaching. These elements include, but are not limited to, developing an identity as a new instructor, preparing for teaching, developing a student clinical assignment, and conducting student evaluation. In this edition, every chapter has been reviewed and content has been updated. There are two new chapters: Chapter 19, "Letters of Reference," and Chapter 20, "Role of Simulation." Chapter 19 identifies the growing importance of recommendation letters written by clinical instructors who have evaluated the clinical performance of students during a practicum experience. Chapter 20 describes simulated learning and explores the increased use of simulation as a learning lab activity. The appendices include sample templates of letters of recommendation plus other valuable and useful material for the clinical instructor. Instructors can preview templates that will assist them with organizing an orientation day, a clinical student assignment, and written assignments. In short, this edition will help you, the clinical nursing instructor, in the role of clinical teacher and will support you in the event you need guidance as you oversee the gradual development of professional caregivers.

Eden Zabat Kan, PhD, RN
Susan Stabler-Haas, MSN, APRN-BC

Acknowledgments

Thank you to all my friends and colleagues for giving me the support and friendship to become the teacher that I am today. This book is dedicated to my parents, Enrico and Edna; you provided me everything that I needed to pursue this career in nursing education. And special thanks to those I truly enjoy working with, Susan Slaninka and Susan Stabler-Haas.

Eden Zabat Kan, PhD, RN

I wish to thank all of my students whose feedback over the years has helped to shape this book. I also would like to thank my husband, Joe. Special thanks to Chris, my son, and my family and friends for all of their encouragement and support. To my co-author, Eden, no one could ask for a better writing partner. Thanks to Susan Slaninka for all her support over the years and for writing the Foreword to our book.

Susan Stabler-Haas, MSN, APRN-BC

Introduction

The major purpose of this book is to provide specific and practical information and guidelines for clinical nursing instructors. Many of these instructors work hard to perform a role, the complexities and frustrations of which are often underrecognized. A clinical instructor has one of the most challenging and potentially rewarding positions in the nursing profession. Today more than ever, it is a role that every state needs to fill in a multitude of programs.

In this chapter, you will read about:

1. The summary of each chapter in this book
2. How the authors intended this book to be used

PURPOSE AND ORGANIZATION OF THIS BOOK

This book has eight major sections and 20 chapters. The chapters provide elemental information applicable to all clinical instructors. Some offer knowledge about the mechanics of clinical instruction, while others assist a new instructor in organizing his or her work. However, this book does not provide all the information necessary to teach student nurses. It is not intended to replace the much-needed graduate programs that focus on teaching registered nurses how to become effective clinical educators. Advanced education focused on the teaching role is highly necessary.

This book is really intended to assist those who have transitioned from the practice role to that of educator. It can serve as a supplemental guide or handbook for those who want to refresh their knowledge about the clinical instructor role.

Parts and Chapters

Part I, which includes Chapters 1 and 2, is an introduction to the clinical instructor role. The first chapter presents the basic facts of clinical teaching and includes the expectations for many novice instructors. In this chapter, you are also asked to assess your knowledge and role. Chapter 2 asks you to assess your basic knowledge of standard rules and policies in nursing education. The chapter also shares information regarding the increased requirements dictated by hospitals prior to entry into their facility.

Part II focuses on the clinical teaching workload. Chapter 3 reviews the priority tasks for the clinical instructor as he or she works not only with students, but also with staff. The chapter also includes a survey of staff nurses, care technicians, and nurse managers regarding their expectations of clinical instructors. Chapter 4 highlights the orientation day and provides a sample template for that day. The orientation day is a key time for communication between the instructor and the students. Tips for fostering student independence and the utilization of a unit "scavenger hunt" are discussed. Chapter 5 discusses the major responsibilities of the clinical instructor's role that will enhance the instructor's relationships with the staff and his or her students.

Part III offers a strategy for maximizing the limited observation and supervision time inherent in the clinical rotation world. That is why many instructors attempt to "see it early."

Chapters 6 and 7 review characteristics of "high fliers" and "not-so-high fliers." High fliers are students who will pass the course and possibly receive a higher than average grade. The "not-so-high fliers" are those who may receive lower grades than most or are at risk for course failure. Strategies to create collaboration between each type of student are delineated, as well as a depiction of the "student's own words."

The key aspects of the clinical evaluation are presented in Part IV. Chapter 8 discusses the importance of student self-evaluation. Students should realize that self-evaluation is a responsibility they will carry into their professional lives as registered nurses. To assist instructors in becoming more efficient in evaluating students, anecdotal note taking is highlighted in Chapter 9 as an advantageous strategy. Chapter 10 provides a more elaborate discussion of warning signs for students who are in danger of failing. Unsatisfactory performance behavior is identified in this chapter as well. Chapter 11 presents the most common grading systems used in nursing programs: letter/number, pass/fail, or satisfactory/unsatisfactory grading systems.

In Part V we reference communication as a key element in most nursing clinical courses. The communication of students is observed in their behavior with patients and in their behavior at group discussion sessions or conferences that take place before and/or after the clinical day. Chapter 12 discusses preconference elements and Chapter 13 focuses on postconferences.

Part VI addresses one of the most difficult challenges faced by the clinical instructor—the assignment of patients to each student. Dealing with unplanned events and their effects on the student–patient assignment is highlighted in Chapter 14. Chapter 15 provides an overview of alternative assignments to optimize the clinical experience of students in any setting.

Part VII focuses on essential competencies found in most programs. Chapter 16 discusses absences and tardiness policies as they apply to the student in clinical rotations. Chapter 17 provides a description of unsafe practice as behaviors not consistent with those documented in the American Nurses Association's Code of Ethics. Safe practice policies are now common in most nursing programs. Finally, Chapter 18 highlights important tips necessary to have a successful and professional relationship with your students and the importance of the instructor's preservation of his or her own health and maintenance of well-being.

This second edition includes Part VIII with Chapters 19 and 20. Chapter 19 discusses the clinical instructor's responsibility regarding writing letters of reference, with sample letters provided in Appendix D. Chapter 20 discusses the current thinking about the utilization of the simulation lab in nursing curricula.

Each chapter includes "Fast Facts in a Nutshell," a feature that highlights key elements of the chapter. Some chapters also provide questionnaires or exercises for you to complete. These are intended to assist in your understanding of the clinical nursing instructor role. Finally, the appendices include several key items that will help you prepare for the role. Items in the appendices are supplemental material for the experienced instructor; however, some novice instructors may find them to be more valuable, especially if they have yet to embark on their first clinical instructor assignment.

DYNAMICS OF CLINICAL INSTRUCTION

As you read each chapter, you will realize the respect the authors have for clinical instruction and the academic goal of providing quality nursing education to future nurses. It is a challenging task to educate a student nurse. We have attempted, in our own way, to provide you—the clinical instructor—with some information about the basic dynamics of clinical instruction. As mentioned earlier, we have years of experience in the role because we truly enjoy it! We commend you for your bravery in embarking on this endeavor.

You should have fun and be open to humor in the role. If you are relaxed, this will be conveyed to your students and will enhance their performance. Moreover, you will quickly realize that there are many surprises in the role. Some students will forward you a "thank you" card at the end of the practicum. Also, do not be surprised if they seek you out at graduation. They may invite you to the final-year, student dinner or the pinning ceremony. Student nurses will become indebted to you and will want to visit you even after graduation from the program. It is a remarkable reward to have that kind of effect on your students.

Lastly, remember the importance of developing a self-care philosophy and practice. Learning how to balance the emotional demands of teaching with your other professional and personal pressures is vital to the art and practice of clinical teaching. Develop your own style of exercise, good nutrition, and "fun." Be a role model to your students by not skipping your meals during clinical, taking some time off from the unit, and practicing self-care.

As your students see you practicing your own self-care, they will realize the importance of imitating your lead. Nursing is a fulfilling and challenging profession. Personal satisfaction is its reward if you practice your own self-care by taking time to meditate, have a hobby, or spend time with family and friends.

Be a role model for your students and you will find much reward in your role as clinical nursing faculty.

You have taken a very important step in your professional nursing career. The fact that you are reading this book shows that you are truly interested in becoming an effective and successful teacher. You have made a commitment to become one of those clinical instructors mentioned in the Foreword by Dr. Slaninka as the one who "made me the nurse I am today!"

You have made a commitment to be an effective clinical nursing instructor.

Congratulations on joining the club!

Appreciating Your New Identity

From Caregiver to Educator

1

Developing a New Identity as a Clinical Nursing Instructor

> *Both novice and experienced nursing teachers need to modify their mindsets on many occasions. They need to shift their actions from the delivery of quality care of patients to the delivery of quality education to students who will one day provide patient care. This chapter introduces the "top 10" facts essential for clinical nursing instruction.*
>
> *This chapter presents a questionnaire for your completion. After answering the questions, you will find explanatory information designed to enhance the development and refinement of your identity as a clinical nursing instructor.*

In this chapter, you will learn:

1. How to begin the transition from staff nurse to clinical nursing instructor
2. The basic facts of clinical teaching

You have just begun a journey from staff nurse to clinical nursing instructor. Or, perhaps, you have been a nursing instructor who always felt the need for more information, more guidance, and more specific examples and plans to successfully instruct your students. Throughout this book, you will learn concrete and useful information that you can use immediately—even on the same day that you read it.

To begin, you should ask yourself two questions:

1. What may be required for my transition from staff nurse to clinical nursing instructor?
2. Which of the following facts do I feel are important?

QUESTIONNAIRE

Place a T for true or an F for false next to the following facts below. Then, review the answers that follow the questionnaire.

_____ 1. I will need to prove my clinical competency on a daily basis.
_____ 2. I will contribute to the nursing profession.
_____ 3. I must be friends with my students.
_____ 4. My students must always like me.
_____ 5. The unit's staff nurses and aides should be happy to take guidance from me.
_____ 6. I want to be familiar with the unit and the staff before I bring my students to the clinical setting.
_____ 7. I must know every detail about every client that my students care for.
_____ 8. I must supervise every procedure and almost all interactions between my students and the patients.
_____ 9. I will earn much more money in this position.
_____10. All of my students will be motivated to learn as much as possible.

ANSWERS TO THE QUESTIONS: TRUE OR FALSE?

1. *I will need to prove my clinical competency on a daily basis.*

    False. Some of you are transitioning from practice as expert staff nurses. Others are tenured professors, academic experts who need additional guidance in supervising students and in grasping the many facets of clinical instruction. Whatever your background, the first item for a clinical instructor to remember is that you will have to supervise clinical experiences with student nurses. The students you will encounter, whether in 2- or 4-year programs, are novice learners. Learning to refrain from performing any nursing skill or procedure for the student learner will be a major challenge. If the student is having a problem performing a basic clean dressing change on a wound, for example, you may be tempted to take over and complete the procedure. Resist taking over! Many seasoned clinical instructors will tell you, "Think more like a teacher and less like a nurse!" Your own professional goals of clinical competence should be tempered. Keep in mind that your role in the clinical setting is to enhance student learning by supervising (and not performing) skills. This involves using teaching and learning strategies to enable the student to perform the clinical skill with knowledge and eventual competence.

    An effective clinical instructor uses these strategies, such as "questioning," "role playing," and "interactive discussion," to improve students' thinking and problem-solving skills. This is not an easy task. Being a good teacher requires much practice and learning.

FAST FACTS in a NUTSHELL

With your students, think of yourself as a clinical teacher rather than a caregiver.

2. *I will contribute to the nursing profession.*

True. Many nurses become clinical instructors without realizing that time is required to transition to the role. Part of the transition is learning the duties and values of that role. According to the American Association of Colleges of Nursing (2001), clinical instructors have, at a minimum, a practice focus and a commitment to decision making and critical thinking pedagogy. The practice of clinical education is highly valued in this current environment of nursing shortages. Whether you are a part-time or full-time clinical instructor, you are contributing to a profession that is in great need of successful instructors who can teach students how to effectively care for their patients.

FAST FACTS in a NUTSHELL

The practice of clinical education is highly valued in this current environment of nursing shortages.

3. *I must be friends with my students.*

False. If you go into clinical teaching thinking that you can be "friends" with your students, then your tenure in this role will be short. As a result of the combined objective and subjective nature of clinical instruction and evaluation, friendships with your students can lead to difficult situations, particularly during evaluation periods. Remember that each school's curriculum establishes many clinical objectives. If you share outside activities with students, you will expend energy that should be focused elsewhere—energy that should be used to enhance your students' clinical competence. In the unfortunate event that you may have to discipline or correct a student under your tutelage, it will be more difficult if you have not maintained the "boundary of teacher:student." Keep personal information about yourself to a minimum.

FAST FACTS in a NUTSHELL

- Maintain the boundary of teacher:student.
- Keep personal information out of the clinical setting.

4. *My students must always like me.*

False. Face it, we all want to be liked as teachers. However, you should first focus on the clinical objectives for your students and place less emphasis on whether students "like" or even "appreciate" your efforts. Wouldn't you rather be the teacher who instills a memorable learning experience? Focus instead on the "aha" moments of your students—moments when your clinical thinking questions led to further student inquiry and successful application of concepts. Once you experience these moments, you will be hooked on teaching. You will realize that friendships and being "liked" cannot replace this feeling of accomplishment.

5. *The unit's staff nurses and aides should be happy to take guidance from me.*

False. Staff personnel, nurses, and aides are familiar with required routines at their clinical agencies and are knowledgeable about their work. Although they are not happy about changes in policy or procedures, they will adapt in time. Thus, they will eventually accept you and your students and be willing to alter their routines a bit. However, they will not be receptive to verbal direction or recommendations from a clinical instructor. If you want to communicate with the staff, ask the nurse manager for the proper procedure.

If, however, a staff member "corrects" you or a conflict develops, try to resolve the issue professionally. Although staff nurses also model professional behavior, you are the daily role model for your students. Remember this when you observe a procedure that is being done incorrectly and you want to provide input based on your practice experience. Recall that you are first a teacher and second a nurse. For those new to the clinical instructor role, this is one of the hardest lessons to learn.

Your major goal as a clinical instructor is to teach your students. You are not there to teach the nurses or other ancillary staff! If you do so, your energy is being misdirected! Instead, direct all your energy to your students. You need some degree of humility. Your goal is to facilitate communication among staff and students, so steer clear of any conflicts. Rather, focus on teaching and preparing your students for success in the practice arena.

FAST FACTS in a NUTSHELL

You are not there to teach the nurses or other ancillary staff.

6. *I want to be familiar with the unit and the staff before I bring my students to the clinical setting.*

True. It is often a prudent practice to go for a "trial run" before you drive to an unfamiliar spot. For example, many people drive to the location of a job interview a day or two in advance to make sure that they know of any detours or potential problems on the route. Similarly, it is vital for any instructor, whether new or familiar with the hospital unit, to visit the unit before the first clinical orientation day with the students. Many hospitals are now being prescriptive with school and clinical faculty requirements. Hospitals and most health care agencies alike will dictate that each clinical faculty entering their agency will either need to: (a) complete a hospital-based orientation, and/or (b) contact the nurse manager of that hospital unit to make arrangements for unit orientation. There are also several documents that need to be submitted to the hospital prior to orientation day. These required documents are similar to what students are expected to submit for entry into clinical practica: current cardiopulmonary resuscitation verification, health requirements, and a background check.

Call the nurse manager and arrange to visit for at least half a day. The nurse manager may meet with you for a brief period, during which you should be prepared to explain the clinical objectives of the course and provide the names of the students with the assigned clinical hours for the term or semester. Also be prepared to ask questions. It is her or his "turf!" You are a guest! Remember that!

You may want to go through a "full shift" with a willing, veteran nurse, thereby becoming familiar with the "culture" and routines of the unit. The bonus is clear: You will have an experienced nurse ally waiting for you when you return with your students.

FAST FACTS in a NUTSHELL

Familiarity with the hospital unit and its staff is an essential element for student learning.

7. *I must know every detail about every client that my students care for.*

False. Remember that the staff nurse is ultimately responsible for the patients, not you! You need to know times of medications, safety information like "code status," NPO (nothing by mouth) status, necessary lab specimens, general diagnoses, and precautions, such as isolation standards. You cannot know all there is to know about the 10 or more patients being seen by the seven or eight students in your group.

Encourage your *students* to assume the responsibility for learning about their patients. It is the student who needs to feel the "pressure" of the obligation to thoroughly read the nursing documentation forms and to check with the primary nurse about the patient. Your job is to foster and encourage the student to gather the client information and remember it throughout the clinical day.

FAST FACTS in a NUTSHELL

Encourage students to be responsible by thoroughly reviewing each patient's chart, medication list, and care plan.

8. *I must supervise every procedure and almost all interactions between my students and patients.*

False. You would be setting yourself up for failure and frustration very quickly if you try to practice this philosophy. While you will need to supervise most medication administration, intravenous medication responsibilities, and new procedures (e.g., insertion of a urinary Foley catheter, insertion of a nasogastric tube, changing of a sterile dressing), you cannot be everywhere all of the time.

In fact, depending on your schedule, you may sometimes allow the staff nurse to supervise your student in putting in a urinary Foley catheter or changing a sterile dressing. For example, you may be supervising one student's administration of intravenous medications when you are notified that another student needs to place a urinary catheter into her patient immediately. If you have established a rapport with the primary nurse whom you believe to be trustworthy and professional, and he or she offers to supervise your student, allow it to happen. You need to trust your staff nurses while broadening your students' experiences.

FAST FACTS in a NUTSHELL

Do not expect to see and supervise each student task.

9. *I will be making much more money in this position.*

False. You may very likely earn less money initially than your graduating seniors do. This is not a lucrative field, except in the area of satisfaction. As we mentioned earlier, when one of your students gets that "aha" moment, it will be worth the pay cut. Remember also that you will be working an academic year, which is only 8 months a year in most settings. You will have opportunities to teach in the summer and develop new courses, which can boost your financial and self-esteem accounts. If you choose to enter the tenured track in an academic institution, your salary will increase incrementally and also more quickly. If you work in an academic institution that has union representation for its professors, this is more likely to be true.

Many opportunities exist to increase your income. You can publish, work as a staff nurse during periods off, consult, and work part-time for one clinical rotation in a different nursing school. All of these expand your horizons. This is an important judgment call for you.

FAST FACTS in a NUTSHELL

Financial gain should not motivate you to become a clinical instructor. Rather, your motive should be to skillfully and effectively teach students to be successful nurses.

10. *All of my students will be motivated to learn as much as possible.*

    False. Sad to say, this is not always the case. Some students will have other life issues that interfere with their ability to devote the time and energy needed to a clinical nursing rotation. Others may not have realized what "nursing" really encompasses and may stay in the major just to graduate and get a job. These students, however, will be in the minority. You will receive satisfaction from the wonderful students who truly are motivated to learn and who will work extremely hard under your guidance. They are the future nurses of whom you will be proud and who will make teaching worthwhile for you. There is no greater satisfaction than to realize that your former students are surpassing you in knowledge—that they have become nurses whom you would want to care for you and for your family.

FAST FACTS in a NUTSHELL

You are helping to educate nurses whom you would want to care for you and your family.

2

Understand the Rules:
What Every Nursing Instructor
Needs to Know About the Nursing
Program's Policies

This chapter discusses the importance of the academic policies at the clinical setting and the specific information that will prove useful to the clinical instructor. The discussion emphasizes that the clinical instructor is responsible for enforcing these policies among his or her students. The chapter begins with a true/false exercise that will enable you to review your baseline knowledge about clinical instruction.

In this chapter, you will learn:

1. Key tasks to be completed by the clinical instructor prior to starting the clinical practicum with students
2. Information that is key to the success of the clinical instructor

Exhibit 2.1   True/False Exercise

For each statement below, check either true or false.

True   False

____   ____   1.   Clinical teaching involves no advance preparation.

____   ____   2.   Familiarity with the nursing program is a priority before your first clinical day with students.

____   ____   3.   The student handbook is one of the most important resources for all clinical instructors.

____   ____   4.   Policies of academic work are not usually found in the student handbook.

____   ____   5.   At the time of hire, you should not expect to receive any written materials about the nursing program.

Answers: 1. False; 2. True; 3. True; 4. False; 5. False

KNOW YOUR BASELINE

Start by answering the true/false questions in Exhibit 2.1. Remember that all clinical instructors must complete a comprehensive examination of their school's nursing program before actually starting the clinical days with students. By the time the instructor is hired, the dean or the nursing program chairperson will probably have supplied a clinical packet that contains essential materials, such as a course syllabus, the faculty handbook, and the student handbook. The instructor is expected to study these materials and return with any questions. It is normal hiring etiquette to provide new clinical faculty with the following:

Essential Clinical Materials

A. Clinical Packet

Clinical Course Syllabus

Clinical Practicum or Academic Calendar Schedule

Clinical Assignment Sheet

Clinical Evaluation Tool (Student and Clinical Faculty)

Diagnostic Medication and Calculation Quiz (a sample copy)

B. Faculty Handbook/Manual

Clinical Job Responsibilities (highlighted)

C. Student Handbook—Clinical Policies

Grading Policy

Dress Code Policy

Attendance Policy

Tardiness Policy

Safe/Unsafe Practice Policy

THE CLINICAL PACKET

The clinical packet is usually a folder of sheets or forms that may include the current course syllabus, an academic calendar or a written outline that highlights the dates of the practicum, and, ideally, certain helpful forms, such as a blank clinical assignment sheet or a copy of a medication quiz (for an example, go to www.alysion.org/dimensional/analysis .htm#problems). This packet also often contains the clinical evaluation tool that will be used to grade each student. As this tool is generally filed in the student's folder at the conclusion of the practicum, be sure you understand how to use it. (For an example of a clinical packet, go to www.dixie .edu/health/nursing/pdfsyllab/1105.pdf.) It is current practice for most nursing programs to offer what is typically called an "adjunct faculty orientation" module. This module will highlight relevant information about the nursing program, faculty and student policies, and other helpful learning modules embedded in an online virtual learning environment. The Des Moines Area Community College has a comprehensive faculty orientation program. You can preview this program online but you will need Shareware/Free software via Adobe Acrobat Reader X or higher (download Adobe Reader from http://www.adobe.com/prodindex/acrobat/readstep.html). To preview the online program, visit http://go.dmacc.edu/ programs/nursing/Documents/Welcome.pdf

THE FACULTY HANDBOOK

If you receive the clinical packet and student handbook without the faculty handbook or a job description, contact the person who hired you. Your program dean or chairperson should refer you to someone who can assist in obtaining necessary information. Most programs have a primary faculty resource for the instructor; they are labeled as a "level or course" coordinator. For example, for a pediatrics course with a related practicum, the pediatrics course coordinator will be assigned to work closely with the clinical faculty regarding student assignments and course requirements. Other programs identify a "level" coordinator or one faculty resource for several clinical practicum courses. In addition, there is a new member of the clinical coordination team. Most nursing programs have now hired a clinical coordinator to further enhance clinical practice coordination among all coordinators. It is a full-time faculty member with relevant experience who may hold a graduate degree in nursing. The clinical coordinator will facilitate communication with the hospitals or health care agencies working with the nursing program. The clinical co-ordinator will provide the clinical packet of information and he or she can assist you in interpreting the clinical evaluation tool, and inform you of any new program updates or changes. Furthermore, your role as a clinical instructor is usually one of an adjunct or "part-time clinical only" faculty member, which means that the position may not require attendance at faculty meetings or certain school functions. In some programs, the information is relayed electronically through email or clearly identified in a job description and in the orientation information that highlights the faculty role. It is the duty of the clinical instructor to keep him-/ herself informed about the student functions of the nursing program. Specific responsibilities and duties are clearly identified in a job description.

STUDENT HANDBOOK

Of all the resources the clinical instructor receives, the student handbook is probably the most valuable and important. In most programs, a student handbook is developed by the faculty in cooperation with students in that nursing program. It is an outstanding resource for all clinical instructors, primarily because it spells out the policies and procedures relating to academic student work. In addition, the handbook contains information about the nursing program and curriculum. It describes not only the program's policies, but also its mission, philosophy, and main goals, as required by accrediting bodies. All nursing schools require accreditation.

Program Goals

Clinical instructors are encouraged to understand the school's goals for its students. There may be times when you are asked to share information about your school with others.

For example, patients or hospital staff may be curious about the school's general program and policies. However, the most important reason to carefully examine the handbook is that it contains explicit instructions for the clinical aspects of the program.

Dress and Attendance Policies

Most health care agencies have policies on everything from dress codes to continuing attendance education. Familiarize yourself with the school's policies because you will be required to enforce them at the clinical site. One that you will need to enforce every day is the dress code! Students must adhere to this dress code, which is usually carefully monitored and evaluated. This code may specify attire, jewelry limitations, hair and nail length, facial piercing, hair color, and other aspects of one's appearance. Adherence to the dress code is identified in a student's clinical evaluation under objectives that specify "professional behavior."

The student handbook also identifies policies on absences, tardiness, and clinical practice expectations. There is usually a zero tolerance for absences or tardiness. Each and every clinical day is considered vital to the overall program. Lateness for the clinical day is always frowned upon. Tardiness and absences are further discussed in Chapter 16.

As mentioned earlier, health care agencies such as hospitals are starting to dictate requirements for clinical faculty that enter their facility. Please check with your hospital site about their specific dress code requirements for faculty. In general, most hospitals prefer clinical instructors to have white lab coats over business attire. For security purposes, they may also require the students and the faculty to wear a hospital-approved identification badge visibly when on their premises.

Program Expectations

Of course, some programs provide more and some provide less information in their student handbooks. Another item that you may find is the clinical practice expectations for each level of the program. In a 4-year nursing program, for example, basic expectations for the second-year student will be different from those for the third-year or fourth-year student. In addition, each clinical site has setting-specific rules and policies; that is, the policies and procedures for a medical-surgical setting will be different from those in the community health clinical rotation. Students will usually receive this information from their clinical instructor at orientation or on their first day at the facility. Chapter 4 provides an outline of the necessary and general information that must be shared with students on orientation day.

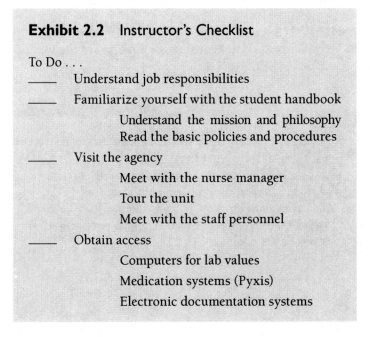

Exhibit 2.2   Instructor's Checklist

To Do . . .

_____ Understand job responsibilities

_____ Familiarize yourself with the student handbook

        Understand the mission and philosophy

        Read the basic policies and procedures

_____ Visit the agency

        Meet with the nurse manager

        Tour the unit

        Meet with the staff personnel

_____ Obtain access

        Computers for lab values

        Medication systems (Pyxis)

        Electronic documentation systems

Yes, most clinical instructors agree that the student handbook is the first item to be reviewed, as it is usually considered the "bible." The novice instructor will probably focus initially on his or her job responsibilities, but the expert will quickly find and read the handbook. To begin the clinical rotation with students and to start planning learning experiences and activities for them, the instructor needs a basic understanding of the school and its student policies. The student handbook is a solid starting place for that information. In addition, the majority of student handbooks are now posted online for public review. For example, refer to the student handbook from the Columbia School of Nursing in New York. Visit http://www.nursing.columbia.edu/students/pdf/StudentHandbook2012-2013.pdf

CLINICAL PRACTICUM

Exhibit 2.2 is an example of a checklist that may help guide what must be done before the first day of the clinical practicum.

FAST FACTS in a NUTSHELL

- Before the clinical practicum begins, make contact with your faculty resource.
- Understand the nursing program's goals and curriculum as highlighted in the student handbook.
- Before orientation day with students, have a clear understanding of the student policies applicable to your clinical course.

Your Success Depends on "YOU":

Preparing for Your Clinical Teaching Assignment

3

You Are a Guest, So Act Like One

Your success depends on "YOU!" This is the first chapter to discuss the essential and "lifesaving" relationship between the clinical instructor and the clinical unit staff. The unit to which you are assigned is NOT a classroom. It is the nursing staff's turf. You are a guest. This chapter provides two examples of novice instructors with different techniques in the clinical setting. You decide whose approach is the more effective and, therefore, the one you should adopt.

In this chapter, you will learn:

1. The art of recognizing the expertise of each nurse and patient care technician and how each one is an expert in his or her domain (even if you disagree with his or her actions)
2. Information and using "EQ" (emotional intelligence quotient) can "make or break" a clinical instructor
3. How to effectively interact with the nursing staff

The clinical site is not an alternative classroom, nor should it be considered the teacher's turf. The clinical site is a nursing unit (or agency) and, therefore, the domain of the nurses who staff it. Your role as clinical instructor does not alter the fact that you are ultimately a guest on their floor or unit. Your goal is to establish the essential and professional "lifesaving" relationship between you and the unit's nursing staff.

The patients for whom the students will care are the responsibility of the unit's staff nurses and technicians. Accede to their sovereignty over patient care. Although rarely discussed in graduate school, this largely unspoken rule is integral to the success of the clinical nursing instructor. Always acknowledge the staff nurses as the experts in rendering care to their patients, even if circumstances may occasionally cause you to question that expertise. There are avenues you can follow if you feel it important to your students' or the patients' welfare to mention a unit nurse's behavior. First, discuss your concerns with the school's coordinator for the course. He or she may have had similar issues in a previous rotation and can give you the benefit of his or her prior experiences. Next, you may need to discuss your concerns with the nursing manager. A word of caution must be given here: Unless a patient's safety is threatened, as a new nursing instructor it is best to pause and seek guidance from either a more seasoned instructor or the school's coordinator before involving the unit's manager with a specific staff complaint. The importance of adopting the proper approach in relating to the nursing staff is illustrated in Exhibits 3.1 and 3.2, which offer two examples of nursing instructors who are about to bring their students into a new unit. You decide which instructor's approach is the more effective.

CASE STUDIES: INTRODUCING STUDENTS TO THE CLINICAL SETTING AND STAFF

Exhibit 3.1   Bob's Approach

Bob is a new hire, eager to begin his first position as a clinical nursing instructor. He has been a critical care nurse for the past 2 years and recently completed his master's degree. He is also new to the facility to which he will bring his first group of students and has called the nurse manager to arrange a meeting with her. He tells the manager that the students will take only patients who are oriented to person, place, and time, and who are able to communicate clearly. He also informs the manager that the students will NOT be helping the clients with their morning care or with any hygiene needs. Bob states, "The students are here to learn their future professional role and that does not include bed making and baths." The manager terminates the meeting abruptly and tells Bob that she thinks there may be a conflict with accommodating his students since a different school of nursing may also be scheduled for the same days. Bob is almost apoplectic, stammering that his students should have priority. The meeting ends badly.

Exhibit 3.2   Mary's Approach

Mary has 5 years of experience as a home health nurse and has two more courses to complete for her master's degree. She has gathered information about the home health agency to which she will soon be bringing her

(continued)

Exhibit 3.2 *(continued)*

students and has arranged to meet with the nurse manager. Mary's students will be working with the agency's nurses and going on home visits with them. Mary explains the objectives of the nursing course to the nurse manager. She details her own experience and acquaints him with the level of expertise of her new students. She requests that the manager tell her which nurses would be most appropriate for the students to accompany on their home care visits. She stresses that the students are prepared to perform many functions under the direct supervision of the professional nurses with whom they are paired. Mary uses the meeting as an opportunity to compliment the nurse manager for allowing students to have this learning experience. Finally, Mary offers to join a nurse herself for one or two visits before the students begin their rotation, so that mutual expectations might be realistically set. The manager arranges for Mary to spend a half-day with one of her more experienced nurses and also states that he will discuss the students' impending arrival at the next agency staff meeting. When he meets with his staff, he intends to highlight the mutual benefits of this professional/student interaction and promises to call back with the names of the nurses who will mentor these students.

Lessons Learned From the Case Studies

Based on these case studies, answer the following questions:

- Which nursing instructor will be successful?
- Which technique received the most positive reaction and feedback?

- Which students will have the best learning experience?
- Which instructor utilized "EQ"?

Unlike Bob, Mary clearly understood that she was a "guest" at the clinical site. She inquired about the agency and apprised the manager about the students' abilities. She asked the manager to assign nurses who really wanted to work with students, thus allowing the staff nurses to have input into the mentoring process. If the members of the nursing staff are given a choice and a voice in teaching (or not teaching) students, it will result in a better experience for the students—and the instructor.

Mary also demonstrated her ability to utilize her EQ. EQ describes an ability or capacity to perceive, assess, and manage the emotions of oneself and of others (Goleman, 1995). She did independent research about the agency, discussed her own expertise and experience, sought the input of the manager, expressed her students' willingness to help the staff, complimented the unit's staff, and extended herself to work with the nurses, seeking their input. As you will see in Exhibit 3.3, Mary included many of the provisions that the nursing staff stated were crucial for nursing instructors to be successful when surveyed.

In conclusion, the rewards from spending at least 1 day (often on your own time) co-assigned with a staff nurse from the new unit where you will be teaching student nurses far outweigh your time investment.

EFFECTIVE INTERACTION WITH THE NURSING STAFF

As is true in any human interaction, understanding the other person's perspective will enhance the chances of a successful outcome. Your hosts in the unit have their own perspectives in terms of their expectations of the clinical instructor and the nursing students. Failure to understand these expectations can lead the unit staff to conclude that you are not fulfilling your responsibility as a guest, even if the omission is quite innocent on your part. The key here is to communicate with the unit staff. So ask: What do they expect from you and the students? Honor their requests when reasonable, and explain the constraints when you and your charges cannot comply. Exhibit 3.3 provides actual comments from two different nursing staffs.

Exhibit 3.3   Informal Survey of Nurses, Patient Care Techs, and Nurse Managers

1. WHAT ARE THE MOST HELPFUL THINGS A CLINICAL INSTRUCTOR CAN DO?
   - Make a list of the students and the patients they are assigned to, and whether they are giving medications that day.
   - Advise the nurse of any issue or change in patient status.
   - Let nurses know what they can help students do.
   - Assign patients to students prior to the staff taking report.
   - Closely monitor the students to ensure that they are not just sitting around.
   - Be present to answer student questions.
   - Help students with medication passes.
   - Be clear about what students are able to do, such as give medications, chart, and so on.

(continued)

Exhibit 3.3 *(continued)*

- Inform staff about the type of patients the clinical instructor is looking for.
- Closely monitor patients that the students are assigned to.
- Ask the patient care technician (PCT) about the unit's morning care routine to avoid confusion.
- Do not allow students to sit in the conference room for most of the shift.

2. UPON ARRIVAL EACH DAY, WHAT INTERACTION OF STUDENTS WITH STAFF IS APPROPRIATE?

- Introduce themselves to the nurse and PCT with whom they will be working, and indicate what they plan to do (bath, medications, vital signs, etc.).
- Give the nurses time to get report from the prior shift before posing questions.
- Accompany the nurse on walking rounds if possible.
- Review available information on the patient's prior night and goals for the day.
- Introduce themselves to each new patient to whom they are assigned.
- Determine whether patients need help eating and whether they are scheduled for tests that day.
- Check the computer for orders.
- Take the patient's vital signs in their first interaction.
- As the day progresses, keep the nurse informed as to what they have done.

(continued)

Exhibit 3.3   *(continued)*

3. UPON LEAVING EACH DAY, WHAT INTERACTION OF STUDENTS WITH STAFF IS APPROPRIATE? WHAT SHOULD THE STUDENTS' FINAL ACTIVITIES BE?

   - Let the staff know when they are done for the day.
   - Do a final set of vital signs before leaving.
   - Give a report of pertinent information, including significant findings and concerns.
   - Document intakes and outputs.
   - Let the nurses and PCTs know what was and was not done.
   - Don't forget to say good-bye to the patients.
   - Inform the nurse if any tasks such as charting have not been completed.
   - Leave the patient comfortable, turning him or her as necessary.

4. OTHER RANDOM THOUGHTS

   - The staff is always grateful to those students who help answer call lights.
   - Students should listen closely when the doctor is in the room, as it is an opportunity to learn.

Note: This informal survey included nurses, PCTs, and nurse managers.

FAST FACTS in a NUTSHELL

- You are a guest; act like one. Positive relationships with the nursing staff are paramount.
- Staff nurses are ultimately responsible for the patients.

4

Organize the Semester—Have a Plan

Instructors are required to review the rules and requirements of the facility where they conduct each clinical rotation. The goal of this chapter is to provide blueprints for the first day of a clinical rotation. Each rotation can last from 4 days to 7 weeks, meeting once, twice, or three times a week. Because each instructor spends most of the first day preparing written expectations and guidelines for students, this chapter presents a template of an orientation day schedule. The sample guides and rules are adaptable to any setting. They have been developed by the authors and used by them quite effectively.

In this chapter, you will learn:

1. How to organize and conduct your first day with your clinical students
2. Which blueprints can be most effectively used with the written guidelines to enhance your students' orientation to the unit and their understanding of responsibilities
3. The benefit of preparing and procuring a signed clinical expectation statement after your orientation day

FIRST DAY OF THE SEMESTER

After your own orientation to the new unit, you can begin to develop your plan for the first day on the floor with your students. Think ahead! You must find a way to communicate to your students when and where you will meet on their first day. After all, the educational experience can be greatly diminished if they don't show up! Here are some possibilities for getting the word out:

- Ask the level coordinator to announce the time and place of the first meeting to your group at the facility, as well as to provide maps and directions online.
- Meet the group members at the school when they have class and provide the same information.
- Use the school's email to provide the initial information.

The goal is to ensure that your clinical group clearly understands the place, time, and attire for the first clinical day. Be clear. Instead of saying, "Meet me in the lobby of the building," be specific. Say, instead, "Meet me in front of the big clock in the Smith lobby at 8 a.m. sharp!" Provide a map with written directions. Don't forget about nourishment. Often this is a 4- to 6-hour day, so inform the students about the lunch possibilities or dinner if you are supervising an evening clinical. Refer to Appendix A for further guidelines to assist you on orientation day.

ORGANIZE

Reserving Space

You must reserve space at the clinical site to conduct your orientation. Most hospitals have a limited number of conference rooms, so you may need to speak with the level coordinator.

However, it is more likely that you, the clinical instructor, will have to obtain that information yourself, either from the nurse educator or the manager assigned to your clinical site.

Whether you will be instructing for 8 days or 8 weeks, *an organized and thorough orientation day will reap dividends* throughout the semester and promote a successful and enjoyable clinical experience for you, your students, and the patients and staff with whom you will be working.

Orientation Day

The first time your clinical group meets should be an orientation day, an evaluation-free period during which instructors show their students the clinical site and clearly explain performance expectations. Students will naturally be anxious during their first few days at your site. If you take a day or even a few hours to review the clinical course and show students where to find certain equipment, their anxieties will ease. Consider using the orientation template that appears on the next few pages. It has been refined and polished over our 30-plus years of clinical instruction. It is adaptable to any setting and any type of nursing program.

Many schools have recently discovered that it is important for students to review essential skills that will be needed in the individual clinical area before the students begin caring for patients. Schools of nursing now email their students weeks before they begin each different clinical rotation and communicate the mandatory review of skills. An example would be to have students review their online modules on tracheostomy care, central venous pressure dressing changes, ventilator care, vital signs, and standard precautions, and complete a questionnaire based on the modules' completion. This questionnaire often needs to be given to the clinical instructor on orientation day. After this preliminary work is completed, it is often expected that each student demonstrate skills such as vital signs procurement, total head-to-toe assessment, therapeutic communication, mental status exam, and tracheostomy care depending on the clinical expectations. Preparations must be part of each orientation to ensure patient safety.

ORIENTATION DAY TEMPLATE

Begin With an Icebreaker

Students often know each other only superficially, if at all. *This makes team building an essential first step.* Your team members must work cohesively if they are to learn the maximum in their short time with you. One example of an icebreaker would be to ask each student to write down on a card two things that the group does not know about him or her. Have each student (including you) choose a card and try to guess which student the card belongs to. You, as the instructor, should also participate in this activity. This will enhance your relationship with your students and help the group members become more comfortable with one another.

Ask Each Student to Define His or Her Goals for the Clinical Practicum Rotation

Collect this information from your students. Give each student a copy of his or her response, and keep one for yourself. If you have this information early in the day, you can better gauge and redefine student expectations. The level coordinator may have given you objectives and goals, but the students may have completely different ideas. If such a discrepancy exists, you need to adjust your orientation by better educating students about the school and the coordinator's objectives. Flexibility is paramount in this role.

Confirm Their Mathematical Competency

If students are administering medications in the clinical practicum, it is prudent to give them a brief and simple medication calculation quiz that requires knowledge of basic math, such as ratio and proportion, and intravenous drip rate equations. Students should be reminded that almost every new registered nurse in a health care facility must pass a medication calculation quiz as a condition of hire. Be sure to acquaint the students with the basic abbreviations used by the institution for the protection of you and the patients. For example, Q.I.D. means 4 times a day, but you should specify what 4 times your institution designates as appropriate, for example, 8 a.m., 12 p.m., 4 p.m., 8 p.m. This cursory evaluation allows you to see if some students need to be sent back to the learning lab for review before they are allowed to administer medications.

Establish the Course Requirements

Like students everywhere, your charges want to know the "bottom line." What do we have to do to pass this clinical rotation? It is a key question, and you should not hesitate to address it. Each clinical instructor brings his or her personality and style to the instruction. The students need to know what you judge as important for their success. Clinical rotations may be pass/fail or result in a letter or numeric grade. All students need a copy of the school's clinical evaluation tool at the outset of the clinical experience, and you should review each line or item with them. Part IV reviews the types of grading systems available in many nursing programs.

Remember, it is your goal to foster independence and safety in each student's clinical experience. Do not hesitate to expect students to arrive early on clinical units to begin their preparation for the day's responsibilities. You do not need to do all of the prep work. Students can arrive early (6:15 a.m.) and talk with the night nurses about patient assignments and gather needed information to present to you in your preconference at 7 a.m. As long as it is established that they cannot go into patient rooms without your presence on the unit and that they are respectful of the nurses' time constraints, this opportunity can foster mutual teaching, connection, and responsibility in your developing nursing students.

Key Components

The following key components must be included in your verbal presentation and in any handouts to students on Day 1, your orientation day.

- The clinical hours that are required; for example, Tuesdays and Thursdays from 7 a.m. to 1 p.m. Wednesdays from 6:30 a.m. to 6:30 p.m.
- The required dates of the clinical rotation. Include any school events or holidays on which there are no clinical days. Establish lines of communication between you and your students and among the students themselves in the event of school closure, and so forth. Will you text, email, call, have a phone chain?—You must address this issue on Day 1.
- The essential expectations that you and the nursing program manager deem most important. For example, attendance and punctuality may be the most basic criteria for assessing performance. If students are not present or not on time, it is difficult to assess performance. Remind them this is all part of their professionalism.
- Contact information should be provided. If the student will be late or absent, how and when do you require him or her to notify you and the unit? If the student needs to contact you at other times during the week, tell him or her the best way, either by email, text, or phone.

- Give sample documentation flow sheets to the students. These are the forms your students will use to write their assessments and notes. If your institution uses electronic charting, first familiarize yourself with this system and then adapt it to your students' needs. Many institutions require that you and your students have completed multiple training modules online to prepare for your role in their institution. Often written evidence of completing these essential modules is required to be given to the manager or nurse educator on Day 1. Find out if each student can receive a password to gain entry into the documentation system as soon as possible—the students will need practice with this skill.
- Journals may also be required. See Appendix B for an instructor's template of written journal requirements.
- Tell your students your policy concerning future written letters of reference (see Chapter 19).
- Prepare and procure a signed clinical expectation statement after your orientation day. See the following example.

CLINICAL EXPECTATIONS SIGNATURE SHEET

[Instructor name] Clinical Rotation for Nsl. 311

I have read [instructor name] guidelines for clinical expectations for ABC Hospital. I have had the opportunity to ask questions about the expectations and I understand the expectations.

_____ (signature)

_____ (date)

Distributed 11/1/20XX

Students' eyes may start to glaze over after about 1 hour of clinical orientation. No matter how interesting and important your information may be, students will gradually lose interest in your "pearls of wisdom." By mentioning that they will need to sign the document shown above at the end of the day, even the most reserved and quiet students immediately discover questions that they urgently need answered. The signed document may also assist you later in the rotation when and if a student asserts that you never told him or her "not to give medications without you." If you have your guidelines and instructions in writing and keep a copy with the student's signed signature sheet, you will have a more successful outcome counseling a student who failed to heed your orientation instructions.

Emphasize the Students' Responsibilities While in the Unit

The nurses in your unit must be confident that your students will properly discharge all their responsibilities before you all leave the unit. For example, if you agree to have the students document a full assessment, perform hygiene care, and administer medication, you must ensure that these tasks are completed before you and the students end the day. If they are not done, the staff will become distrustful and disinclined to allow you or your students to care for their patients. They may also hesitate to teach and share knowledge with your students. One fact cannot be overemphasized—*the instructor's relationships with the staff and nurse unit manager are paramount for a successful clinical experience* for the students and for the instructor. Post a written guide to the staff of the student's responsibilities while on the unit.

Take the Tour

At the beginning or end of orientation day, the instructor may schedule a visit to the unit. If you arrange this visit at the end of the day, remember that students may have already reached their saturation point for absorbing information. You may only be able to give them a handout with essential codes to use to gain entry into kitchens, utility rooms, and medication rooms. The handout can include a sample schedule of their clinical day or a list of their patients (see Appendix C for a sample student schedule). Another suggestion is to let the students review a patient chart and have them walk around and tour the unit on their own. Many nursing instructors distribute a "scavenger hunt" guide (see Exhibit 4.1) for the students to use during their initial orientation tour on the unit.

Exhibit 4.1   Scavenger Hunt for XYZ Skilled Nursing Facility

Please find the following and jot down where you found each item. If the hunt involves a person, note the name and any information that might be helpful for our group. We will discuss your results at postconference today.

1. Clean linens to change a bed
2. Clean washcloths and towels
3. The makings for tea or coffee
4. The dining area and who eats at each dining room
5. The residents' personal toothpaste, deodorant, soap, etc.
6. Residents' charts
7. The latest record of their medications
8. The nurse who is caring for your resident (remember your own introduction—name and school)
9. The nurse's assistant who is caring for your resident (remember your own introduction)
10. Location of thermometer, pulse oximeter, blood pressure measurement device

(continued)

Exhibit 4.1   *(continued)*

11.   Unit secretary (remember your own introduction)
12.   Location of residents' clothing

This is a good start. Feel free to record anything else that you learned and all questions noted as you complete this sheet.

FAST FACTS in a NUTSHELL

- Be organized and have a plan for orientation day.
- Provide detailed written information and distribute a copy to students.
- Ensure that all student responsibilities are completed before leaving the unit each day.

5

Confidentiality and Patient Privacy

Use discretion always. In other words, do not talk about patients in the elevators, in public spaces, or in front of individuals not specifically designated by the patient to receive information. This chapter provides specific examples of students who violated patient privacy by speaking "innocently" about their patients outside of the clinical setting. Information will be given about maintaining patient privacy while delivering care in the unit.

In this chapter, you will learn:

1. Relevant provisions of the Health Insurance Portability and Accountability Act (HIPAA) and how it interfaces with your students
2. Ways in which students can violate patient privacy
3. Basic suggestions to avoid violations of privacy

CONCEPTS OF CONFIDENTIALITY
AND PATIENT PRIVACY

The concept of confidentiality in health care enjoys widespread acceptance in the United States. Maintaining the confidentiality of client health care information is both a legislative and professional imperative, as underscored by the Health Insurance Portability and Accountability Act of 1996 (HIPAA) and the American Nurses Association (ANA) Code of Ethics. HIPAA was designed to increase the confidentiality of patient information.

Students may be on the same units as their neighbors, peers, or family and friends. It cannot be emphasized enough that absolutely *no* information about any client/patient can be discussed with anyone outside of the unit's perimeter. When a breach occurs, litigation can follow.

Teaching the Concepts

Most nursing programs teach the concepts of patient privacy and confidentiality in the classroom as part of their Fundamentals course, as it is considered "essential" knowledge prior to beginning any clinical practicum rotation. Your students may have been informed about HIPAA and the legal implications of not protecting patient information, but the actual practice of enforcing patient privacy in the clinical field is another matter. As a nursing instructor, you must educate your students and monitor their discussions to ensure that the privacy of each client is protected. Never hesitate to impress upon these future practicing nurses how this is a vital function of their role and a nursing duty as highlighted in the ANA's Code of Ethics (ANA, 2001).

The goal is to apply the theory taught on HIPAA to the clinical field. That is, the clinical instructor must ascertain the degree of student understanding and, most importantly, how HIPAA requirements apply to the clinical setting. In an acute care setting, for example, there are multiple times when students may encounter visitors at their patient's bedside. They have to be careful to whom they speak and what information they convey to these visitors. There have been occasions on which visiting family and neighbors received health information that they should not have been given.

CASE STUDIES

The case studies in Exhibits 5.1 and 5.2 present two different scenarios that emphasize the need for each instructor to stress daily to students that *client confidentiality is paramount.*

As these cases demonstrate, the aphorism that encourages the "ounce of prevention" rings especially true in the clinical setting. One must also emphasize the need for privacy while on the unit itself. This means that all computer screens must be turned off when students are not using them. If a visitor simply walks past an unattended computer screen and inadvertently sees patient information, a violation of privacy has occurred and liability could possibly result for those nurses on the unit.

Exhibit 5.1 Hannah's Scenario

During Hannah's geriatric rotation, she cared for an 80-year-old patient. She did an excellent job and was complimented by her instructor and by the staff. She went home and told her family how much she enjoyed caring for her client and what happened during her day. She mentioned the patient's name to her family, thinking that he lived in a different town and that no one could possibly know him. Based on the circumstances

(continued)

Exhibit 5.1 *(continued)*

of the patient's case, the student's mother correctly concluded that the patient was in fact the father of one of her employees. This worker had missed a lot of time lately supposedly because of personal illness. She became angry that her employee was not ill as she had claimed, but rather was taking time off to be with her father. The student was very concerned that her mother would reprimand the staff member, causing the employee to subsequently question how the mother had obtained this information. The student now wondered if she needed to inform her nursing instructor of the confidentiality breach.

Exhibit 5.2 Grace's Scenario

Grace had to present her client to her clinical group and was preparing the presentation in her dormitory room. She had her patient's name on all of the information that she was preparing and left the presentation material on her desk. Later in the day, her former high school friends came to visit and planned to stay overnight in her room. One friend read the information on her desk and exclaimed that the patient was her boyfriend's mother. She also said that her boyfriend does not live with his mother and was not aware of his mother's clinical psychiatric situation. She began to call him on her cell phone to inform him that his mom was in a psychiatric facility. Grace pleaded with her to not call and tried to explain how she would be in serious trouble if this information about the client was revealed.

FAMILY MEMBERS

Another potential problem involves the information that you may share with family members of the patient. It is the patient—not the health care provider—who controls the disclosure of health information. You must *procure the patient's permission* before you can discuss his or her medical condition with the family. If family members are present in the room and the client asks you questions, you are still on somewhat shaky ground. It is prudent to discuss with clients beforehand what information they want discussed and shared with family members. If you have any doubts, ask the family to briefly leave the room and then ask the client to clarify what areas are acceptable to discuss. You can also ask the client to sign a consent form before the discussion takes place, especially if sensitive material is to be discussed. Information about AIDS, sexually transmitted diseases, substance abuse, and psychiatric illness are considered especially sensitive.

FAST FACTS in a NUTSHELL

- Always use discretion concerning client privacy.
- No information should be divulged without consent.
- Before sharing information with families, confer with patients.

PART

III

Getting to Know Your Nursing Students

Who Are the Best and Who Are the Rest?

6

The High Fliers: How to Screen for Higher Achieving Students

One of the challenging aspects of clinical teaching is managing students during the limited blocks of time available for instructor observation. Practicing nurses work 8- or 12-hour shifts, whereas student nurses are usually at the clinical sites for 4- to 8-hour blocks of time. As a result, many clinical instructors try to see things "early." That is, most seasoned clinical instructors try to identify or classify their students within the first week of the clinical rotation. One such classification would be students "at risk" (at risk of failing the course) and students "not at risk."

In this chapter, you will learn:

1. The characteristics of students who are not at risk, those who are considered "high fliers"
2. The advantages of classifying students early in the program

ASSESSING STUDENT CAPABILITIES

The clinical instructor is first and foremost a teacher. To become an effective teacher, the instructor must assist students to learn to problem solve and think at a higher level. Therefore, the successful instructor needs to develop quick insight into the nature and capabilities of the students. Within the first 2 weeks of the clinical rotation, the instructor should be able to distinguish between the high fliers, those who will potentially receive higher grades, and the not-so-high fliers whose success cannot be immediately assured.

IDENTIFYING THE HIGH FLIERS

This distinction is also important because the clinical instructor faces certain stresses when dealing with a student who is at risk of failing the clinical course. The first sign of possible failure is unsatisfactory behavior when performing a nursing skill. The instructor needs to take extra time to manage this behavior while continuing to teach the other students within the time frame set by the nursing program.

Surprisingly, for some instructors, identifying the high fliers is quite easy. Some use instinct. For example, some students may impress you by completing homework earlier than the rest of the group or by earning a high grade on the medication quiz. Sometimes a student's question may give you an impression of that student's cognitive ability. For example, one student may ask, "I just took vitals on my patient. What do I do next?" In comparison, another student may voice, "I took vitals on my patient. Now I am starting the nursing assessment because I plan to give the medications soon." Obviously, the second student has a clear understanding of the nursing process and can initiate interventions competently. Initiating interventions competently is a major objective for student nurses, as it is a basic requirement and goal of graduation. This goal, as well as other goals for students, is usually documented in the student handbook of most nursing programs.

CHARACTERISTICS OF HIGH FLIERS

Based on years of experience and bearing witness to all kinds of student behaviors, the following are the most common characteristics of high fliers.

1. *The student is prepared each clinical day and displays this during the clinical rotation.*

   This student has reviewed his or her patient assignment and has some knowledge base to share with you about the patient's condition. If assigned to give medications that day, he or she will have medications reviewed and written down. This student may even present you with pages of written or typed notes of the work he or she did in preparing for the clinical day. Those papers will include information about the patient's medical disease process and the management of the medications. Each medication the patient is prescribed may be documented. The student will also bring his or her own books to the clinical facility.

2. *The student communicates well orally with you and the patients.*

   This student asks you questions about the patient and can clearly verbalize some information about the assigned patient. When observed, this student is comfortable at the bedside speaking to the patient and the staff nurses. The student may show initiative by, for example, using the Internet to research topics like smoking cessation or dietary needs, such as foods that are high in fiber.

3. *The student prioritizes patient interventions appropriately.*

   For example, in a medical-surgical dayshift rotation, without your direction you witness the student rechecking a heart rate because the patient complained of dizziness.

Another example is, at a community rotation, the student may check the vital signs and promptly report to you or the staff nurse an abnormal blood pressure and heart rate. This student may even ask a staff nurse to recheck the vital signs with him or her for accuracy.

FAST FACTS in a NUTSHELL

- It is best to distinguish the high fliers early.
- High fliers are prepared, communicate at a higher level, and can prioritize nursing interventions better.

7

The Not-So-High Fliers:

How to Screen for Potential "Problem Students"

Teaching in the clinical setting requires an enormous amount of preparation before the course begins and then prior to each clinical day. One major frustration for instructors is the limited time available at the clinical site to teach all the students. In some acute care settings, the student-to-instructor ratio is a surprising 10:1. State boards of nursing are well aware of this fact. One practice that can assist the clinical instructor is the early identification of strong students (high fliers) and weak students (not-so-high fliers). Often, you as the instructor can strategize ways for the high fliers to assist and provide needed role modeling for the not-so-high fliers.

In this chapter, you will learn:

1. The characteristics of the not-so-high fliers
2. How to compare high fliers and not-so-high fliers
3. Strategies to assist the not-so-high fliers

IDENTIFYING AT-RISK STUDENTS

Instructors need to "see it early" according to Teeter (2001). That is, they need to identify the at-risk students or the not-so-high fliers by certain "red flags." Some of these red flags are: "The student arrives late on the first or second day," or the student is "unengaged with learning" or the student "frequently gets staff and other students to help" (Teeter, 2001, p. 91). Sometimes, you may at first think that some students have really good relationships with the staff of nurses, nurse assistants, and technicians, particularly as you witness their close interactions. But this can be a warning sign. It is wise to keep an extra careful eye on these students just to make sure that they are doing their work and not just "copying" data from what has already been documented. They could even be getting answers to your questions from the staff nurses!

"Seeing it early" is a good strategy to employ as a clinical instructor. The not-so-high fliers may be more difficult to notice. Develop a keen sense of awareness. For example, some instructors might automatically stigmatize students who stay at the patient's bedside or are difficult to find during the clinical day. However, these students may not be at risk. Yes it's true that students who are nowhere to be found may be "hiding" from you and your questions about their patient's care, but that student may also just be spending time caring for his or her assigned patient and being extremely attentive to the needs of that patient. You need to discern these differences.

CHARACTERISTICS OF NOT-SO-HIGH FLIERS

Here are a few characteristics of the not-so-high fliers and a discussion of each, which are listed in Table 7.1.

1. *The student is not thoroughly prepared each clinical day.*

    In most cases, there is a great deal of self-directed preparation on behalf of the student. Not-so-high fliers, however, will be unprepared even though they may have

TABLE 7.1 High Fliers Versus Not-So-High Fliers

High Flier	Not-So-High Flier
1. Prepares for each clinical day	1. Does not thoroughly prepare for the clinical day
2. Communicates clearly with instructor and/or patients and staff nurses	2. Inconsistent with communication (e.g., may not have verbalized to you an abnormal vital sign)
3. Prioritizes patient interventions appropriately	3. Unsure about patient care priorities

been instructed to prepare for a particular procedure, such as Foley catheter insertion or medication shot. Another example is assigned written work. Whatever the case, the not-so-high fliers will not turn in their work or will turn in work that is incomplete.

Whether the assignment is written or oral, the not-so-high fliers will have an excuse as to why their performance is not up to par and why they are "unprepared." More likely than not, the clinical instructor will witness such a student sitting in the back of a nursing lounge with an open textbook, writing down the information that he or she should have arrived with at the beginning of the clinical day. This student may also be observed in clandestine discussion with more prepared fellow students in an apparent attempt to obtain answers to questions that you have previously posed to this not-so-high flier.

2. *The student is inconsistent in communicating information (e.g., the student may not have informed you of a patient with a high blood pressure [BP] value).*

The not-so-high fliers are less assertive than the others in the group. That is, they are more comfortable being spoken to than actually initiating a conversation with you! As a result, they may not convey information promptly. They may know they are hearing something abnormal in the lungs or note a higher BP value in a patient, but they cannot decide what the next step should be. They do not speak to the staff nurse or a fellow student to seek their feedback. In fact, instead of speaking to anyone about their suspicions, they keep the information to themselves.

The instructor should allow for the possibility that inadequate communication may be the result of inherent shyness and not a lack of knowledge or preparation. Therefore, the instructor must do some careful probing before judging the student's potential. Although students who are shy may avoid eye contact or nonverbal behavior, this does not necessarily mean they are not-so-high fliers. Further questioning of the student in a private place or at your office may be warranted to gain a bit more understanding of the student. Taking away part of the anxiety (being in the role of a clinical student during a clinical performance day) may actually help you to get more insight into your student.

3. *The student is unsure about patient care priorities.*

Every clinical rotation has expectations of basic student competencies and skills. It is expected that students advance through each rotation and make improvements within a given clinical rotation. This is most true in medical-surgical settings where nurses care for multiple patients with various medical needs. Nurses are taught to prioritize their actions. They learn this skill during clinical rotations with clinical instructors.

The not-so-high fliers struggle with prioritizing basic care for their patients. To them, every intervention is a priority. A morning bath may be more important than getting the morning vital signs. Providing the evening snack as soon as it arrives may be more important than checking if the patient is diabetic and needs insulin first. They may not know that assessment of heart sounds is a priority action before administering a prescribed beta blocker medication. This problem with prioritization may either be a thinking problem or a problem related to self-induced anxiety. For example, a patient may have just woken up and asked the student to set up a bath. Not thinking through the care tasks for the day, the student happily helps the patient get this done before all other assessments.

MONITOR NOT-SO-HIGH FLIERS

Once you have some idea of which students are the not-so-high fliers in your clinical group, keep a critical eye on them. That's it! It is also wise to be attuned to comments from staff nurses about these students. If these students are not performing their required duties, you will hear about this from the nursing staff (especially if you have developed a collegial relationship with them). As noted in Chapter 3, students and the clinical instructor are guests in the unit. Thus, any tasks not completed by the student will be reported by the staff personnel to the nurse manager, who will then immediately notify you. Many instructors are not happy receiving a phone call about a missed task. Therefore, communicate clearly and early with your students about their responsibilities.

Another word of caution about the not-so-high fliers. They may also be those students who are habitually late in leaving the clinical site. That is, at the end of the clinical day, students usually gather at one spot to walk to their conference site for postconference, or they independently meet at a designated time and location for postconference. The at-risk student may lag behind one day and then the next and then the next. When it happens once, try to get the cause for the lateness—maybe a patient had an unexpected test or, for a home visit, maybe the client was unavailable. If it happens repeatedly, it is a cause for concern. A similar finding for this student is that he or she may be the one that other students gather around. This may just be a casual student gathering, but this can also mean that the not-so-high flier has asked for and is receiving assistance from peers in answering questions.

One strategy that has great benefits for both high fliers and not-so-high fliers is pairing one student from each category and giving specific guidelines for this intervention. You can make this part of your total clinical experience and expectation for your rotation.

For example, select one student from each flier category who will then collaborate as a two-person team. Of course, you will avoid any mention of your categories or your reasoning for the pairing. Have them work together to provide care for a group (two to four) of patients. One student will be the "professional nurse" and the other the nurse's patient care tech. It is the responsibility of the nurse to gather all information, communicate this to his or her team, procure or provide all needed care and information to the patients, communicate to the primary nurse, and do all of the reporting and documentation. These two roles should be reversed on the next clinical day with the same two students. Have the high flyer be the professional nurse on Day 1 of the experience, and the not-so-high flier assume the same responsibility on Day 2.

Here is the reaction of one student who participated in this role-sharing clinical experience:

> It was my first time pairing up with a partner and to experience team work, management, and delegation. Through this experience I once again learned about the crucial aspect of communication within a team. I was really grateful that I had the chance to work with another peer because it allowed me to delegate roles such as obtaining vital signs and communicating, which was crucial because my patients were on meds that required taking a blood pressure or a pulse.

Don't forget to explain the above strategy to the staff on the unit ahead of time so they are aware of which student is responsible for each patient's needs.

Lastly, one of the most useful tools or strategies any clinical instructor can utilize is to co-assign the student with a "willing" staff nurse. Basically, you first need to establish your collegial relationship with the staff, then discuss the possibility of having your students (one by one) work alongside a primary nurse for the shift. Develop goals and objectives of the experience for the students to document along with their feelings and thoughts at the completion of the shift. The following are some comments from senior students after they spent a shift with a primary staff nurse:

> I really learned a lot from Kerry. It was amazing to see how good of a nurse she was, and how much she learned along the way just from practicing. It made me feel a bit more comfortable about the process of graduating and starting my experience as a real nurse. She taught me a lot of time-management skills, precision, detail-oriented skills, and how to accomplish everything you want to during a shift in a concise manner.

> Following Edie was such a great learning experience. It made me a little bit stressed out about all of the responsibilities of a nurse. I realized how organized I will have to be, and how important each and every task is, and how essential it is to be aware and present while you are working. These are not new ideas to me but this shadowing experience made it all that much more real. It also made me very excited to graduate and be independent!

If you need extra help monitoring some of the students, ask the staff. Seeking the staff's input is always a wise move, as it may or may not validate the traits that you see in the student. More frequently, though, the staff will come and inform you who they think are your higher-level students. Unsolicited feedback about your students is a normal aspect of the clinical teaching arena.

To summarize, if you spot a not-so-high flier in your clinical group, just keep an eye on that student! No further action is needed on your part. You will be too busy with the normal day's tasks to do anything else with these students, unless of course, a problem occurs. The instructor may continue to observe unsatisfactory behavior. If you are seeing more "red flags" and are unsure about them, review Chapter 10. If more than one "flag" is identified, the instructor is now warned that the student is in jeopardy of clinical course failure. A more elaborate listing of these behaviors is identified in Chapter 10.

FAST FACTS in a NUTSHELL

- Not-so-high fliers may be difficult to spot.
- High fliers can sometimes augment your own efforts in helping the not-so-high fliers improve their performance.
- Be open to the staff's input regarding certain students.

PART

IV

The Performance Appraisals

Clinical Evaluations

8

Making the Most of Student Self-Evaluation

In some programs, students are required to rate their own performance based on the objectives set by the program or the clinical instructor. Students may need assistance in understanding how to effectively complete a self-evaluation. These evaluations are important, as they provide the nursing instructor with a blueprint to use in communicating concepts to students, who in turn will be better prepared to accurately assess their own performance.

In this chapter, you will learn:

1. The nature and purpose of student self-evaluations
2. Suggestions for the instructor to use in guiding students toward a realistic evaluation

63

STUDENT PERFORMANCE EVALUATION

One of the most important aspects of clinical care coordination is evaluation (Potter & Perry, 2013). This principle logically extends to evaluation of care rendered by nursing students. Careful explanation of the clinical evaluation tool, including specific examples, should occur at the outset to clearly establish the expectations you will have of your students as they navigate through their clinical experiences. Emphasize to your students that performance evaluations will be an ongoing process throughout their nursing careers.

EVALUATION PROCEDURES

Once hired by the nursing program, your initial orientation to the clinical instructor role should include a detailed explanation of the procedure used to evaluate each student's clinical performance. This is comparable to the first day in the traditional classroom, when the teacher reviews the course syllabus and details the method by which the course grade will be determined. Various nursing clinical evaluation tools involve "grading." Others are based on the "pass/fail" model. Chapter 11 describes the differences and the challenges of both models, along with examples of each.

STUDENT SELF-EVALUATION

Regardless of what type of evaluation tool is employed, most nursing programs require students to perform a self-evaluation. Usually, students submit their self-appraisal a few days before the planned evaluation from the instructor. Senior students with 6 or more days of clinical instruction may also be required to submit a self-evaluation for their mid-term.

A mid-term evaluation enables the instructor to recognize good performance and facilitate remedial action where needed. Refer to the "Early Warning System" (Chapter 10) for a more detailed explanation of the merits of a mid-term evaluation.

According to Gaberson and Oermann (2010), development of self-evaluation skills is paramount for nurses. Because nurses must be competent in a practice that involves daily management of patients' illnesses and the skillful use of pharmacological therapies and life-saving equipment, it is essential that nurses continuously self-monitor their performances. Throughout their careers, nurses must determine when they need more education or skill training. It is important, therefore, to foster the development of self-evaluation skill in the student nurse.

Exhibit 8.1   Student Self-Evaluation of Clinical Performance

Grading Methodology
Grading for performance at the clinical site will follow the (*course name or number can appear here*) evaluation tool.

This self-evaluation is your opportunity to comment on your clinical performance. The grade range is a 1 to 5 Likert scale, which is defined as follows:

      1 – Does not meet clinical criteria

      2 – Is inconsistent in meeting clinical criteria

      3 – Meets clinical criteria

      4 – Exceeds clinical criteria

      5 – Far exceeds clinical criteria

(*continued*)

Exhibit 8.1 *(continued)*

Example Objective
"Attend each clinical session and submit required materials."

If your daily performance and submitted materials meet the expected standard, you may assign yourself a 3. If you exceed these minimum requirements, you may award yourself a 4 or 5, but you must provide *written* evidence for this elevated grade. Keep a log of any instances where you performed above minimum criteria. You cannot rate yourself higher than a 3 if you do not provide the written evidence for that grade. Submit this evidence with your self-evaluation. In the context of this example, here are some ways to exceed clinical criteria and achieve a grade above 3:

- Arrive on the unit early to read your client's chart and to ask pertinent questions at the 7 a.m. preconference.
- Submit more than the minimum requirement of one journal per week. Incorporate classroom objectives and knowledge.
- Present a clinically related topic of interest to peers or a client.
- Conduct independent research regarding your client's care.

Note: Self-evaluation grades higher than 3 that are not supported with written evidence of accomplishment will be reduced to 3.

SAMPLE GRADING METHODOLOGY

The sample student evaluation grading methodology illustrated in Exhibit 8.1 can be shared with your students on the clinical orientation day. This example is suited for clinical evaluations that are in a graded format. Many students report that the process of self-evaluation can be anxiety provoking. Although this may be true, mild anxiety can promote personal growth. The discussion that ensues once the instructor examines, reviews, and responds to the student's self-evaluation can be invaluable. It teaches the student how to accept constructive criticism and provides specific feedback and data on his or her performance. If a mid-term evaluation is possible, an action plan can be developed for the remainder of the course.

Many students are seeking feedback and suggestions in their ongoing pursuit of competency in clinical nursing. This evaluation time can be one of the most important sessions of their entire nursing curriculum. Many of today's experienced nurses can cite an instance when a clinical instructor gave them positive or negative feedback during a clinical evaluation and the impact of that situation on their nursing careers.

FAST FACTS in a NUTSHELL

- Student self-evaluation is a valuable tool.
- Guidelines that instruct students how to document their performances are recommended.
- Students' self-evaluations, when compared with the instructor's assessment, are important opportunities for dialogue and feedback.

9

The DO's and DON'Ts of Student Documentation

A common mistake that clinical instructors make in their student clinical evaluations often involves insufficient documentation. "Anecdotal notes" are useful as the traditional format to document clinical performance. However, more official documentation by the clinical instructor becomes imperative when the student's performance leaves him or her in jeopardy of not passing the course. This chapter illustrates examples of anecdotal notes. It also offers concrete directions on the type of data needed to document the evaluation in a timely way.

In this chapter, you will learn:

1. How to document "anecdotal notes"
2. Key aspects of documentation pertinent to the clinical instructor

DOCUMENTING STUDENT PERFORMANCE

The clinical instructor's assessment of student performance is an ongoing process. The student's evaluation should reflect a compilation of these observations. Ensuring that the student evaluation presents a fair picture of performance requires avoiding common mistakes of judgment.

THE DON'TS

As a new instructor:

- DO NOT adopt a casual approach to documenting a student's clinical performance.
- DO NOT depend on "remembering" the specifics of each student's experiences when: (a) administering medications, (b) assessing clients, (c) teaching clients, and (d) interacting with staff, their peers, or even with you!
- DO NOT think that because the student is hanging an intravenous medication or inserting a urinary catheter for the first time, mistakes should be disregarded because of a lack of preparation.
- DO NOT conclude that little harm or injury will ensue after a student encounter, such as patient assessment, even though the nurse stated that the client was "upset" that day.
- DO NOT assume that the instructor has no financial or legal risk associated with student errors because students carry their own liability insurance.

THE DO'S

Be cautious. Too casual of an approach to documenting a student's clinical performance can lead to a final student evaluation that cannot be supported. The instructor may "feel" that a student adequately performed during a specific clinical rotation, but did not exceed the minimum expectation of the clinical program. That student may, quite possibly, have an entirely different perspective. The student may believe that he or she performed in an exemplary manner and can cite specific examples in his or her self-evaluation. Unless the instructor has maintained an organized file of "anecdotal notes" to refute this perception, the instructor's assessment may face a student challenge that can often involve extensive follow-up and work by the instructor.

This may include discussions between the instructor and the level or course coordinator or school chairperson, as well as other assigned faculty members. There are usually procedures in place regarding these types of student issues. Each nursing program has a different procedure for handling student clinical course issues.

If an instructor depends on "remembering" the specifics of each student's experience, the student evaluation can be murky and irrelevant. With a number of students to evaluate, even a person with a sharp memory may have difficulty recalling the specifics of each student's performance, including the adequacy and degree to which various nursing skills were implemented and evaluated.

In evaluating students, never disregard "lack of preparation." If students have been notified that they will be administering medications and performing certain procedures, it is incumbent upon the students to prepare by practicing in the nursing lab. Clinical instructors often have minimal time to teach and review an entire procedure for a student, particularly if the client is to receive treatment in a timely manner. Nursing labs are available in all nursing programs today. Many labs have actually been revised and updated to incorporate high-fidelity simulation experiences (see Chapter 20 for more information). It is the students' responsibility to make arrangements to visit the lab and review necessary skills before their clinical experiences.

Make the nursing staff your ally. They have eyes and ears that can interpret and gather more information about your students' performance than you can obtain alone. If a staff nurse or nursing assistant mentions to you that a patient or the family seemed upset after the student performed a skill or entered a client's room, *investigate.* This revelation often is a "red flag" that indicates a possible problem for the student, the school of nursing, and *you.* Go into the patient's room, introduce yourself to the patient and family, and ask how the student interaction was received by the client. It is better to take care of any potential problem immediately rather than let it fester. Addressing it a week or two later may mean the difference between a prompt resolution and a legal situation.

Another helpful tip is to check with the nurse manager from time to time. This is being proactive as a teacher and evaluator. Go and inquire if there have been any concerns or issues. You may hear issues from patients or staff that fell through the cracks. However, checking in with the nurse manager will enhance your relationship with him or her, and often earn the goodwill of the nursing staff as well. When the nursing program submits its routine inquiries to clinical sites requesting placement for the uncoming semester, that unit will ask for you!

FINANCIAL LIABILITY

Understand your financial liability at the clinical site. Teachers and students are held to the same standards of care that a reasonably prudent person with the same level of education and experience would use in the same or similar circumstances (Oermann & Gaberson, 2009). Teachers are not liable for negligent acts performed by their students if they have done the following:

1. Selected appropriate learning activities based on skills necessary to complete the assignment.
2. Determined that the students have the necessary knowledge and skills to complete the assignment.
3. Provided necessary guidance.

Yes, your students do have liability insurance, but you too are liable if the aforementioned standards are not in place when your student performs an unsafe act. As an instructor, it is prudent to carry liability insurance. Check with national nursing organizations, which can provide further information about liability insurance for educators. You can also check with the chairperson or head of your nursing program for this information. Many schools of nursing require that you show evidence of malpractice insurance when you are first hired.

ANECDOTAL NOTES

Each day, the instructor will have students assume an assignment (as detailed in Part VI). It is helpful for the clinical nursing instructor to devise a system for maintaining "anecdotal notes" relating to each student's performance. Your own notes during the day will help jog your memory when it is time to conduct the clinical evaluation. You may also want to maintain a book with a separate page for each student—a copybook of sorts. After each clinical day, jot down a few notes about each student. An example of such a note might be:

> Mary administered Ancef IV and gave three oral medications to her patient. Her knowledge base of the oral medications was weak. I recommended to her that she write down pertinent facts about the meds before she contacts me saying she is prepared to give meds.

Writing such brief notes will help you identify whether a specific student followed your suggestion or repeated the same weak performance the next time that she was assigned to administer medications. If a particular student repeated the same substandard performance, it could be a "warning" sign. Discussion of warning signs for clinical instructors can be found in Chapter 10.

It is also helpful to keep a log of your comments regarding any written work submitted during the clinical practicum. For example, if weekly journals are due, devise a system to rate the journals and either write a number on each assignment or write your own note for each assignment in your own anecdotal notes. Thoughts like "needed much prompting on written journal in week 2 to include all categories of med classifications" will suffice to support your grading later in the semester. Check in with the level or course coordinator regarding any written assignments. They may also have a grading rubric or grading form that can assist with the overall evaluation of the assignment.

Any system for keeping notes will do. Even an electronic record of this information is effective. The bottom line is that you need to write a note or two on each student each day of the clinical rotation, so take the time to document. The nursing profession teaches new students that if it is not documented, it did not happen. For a successful student evaluation, make sure that your anecdotal notes reveal what did happen.

FAST FACTS in a NUTSHELL

- Avoid the "mistakes" of a new clinical instructor by documenting student performance.
- Anecdotal notes are paramount for all instructors.
- Written recordings of clinical performance are needed to support documenting a student's weakness or failure.

10

Early Warning System

Many experienced clinical nursing instructors use a large amount of intuition when observing students. There are usually warning signs if a student is in jeopardy of not meeting the clinical objectives of the course. For example, a student may perform a nursing skill in a certain manner or communicate an aspect of the nursing process in such a way that the experienced instructor is alerted to a potential problem. Because nurses are charged with serious and potentially life-sustaining responsibilities, these sometimes subtle "warning signs" are important to heed and address.

In this chapter, you will learn:

1. How to identify the warning signs that a student may be in jeopardy of not passing or safely performing in the clinical setting
2. Important tips to develop a "sixth sense," or intuition, to help determine which students are at risk for performing unsafe practices on patients

EARLY WARNING SIGNS

As stated in Chapter 8, a mid-term evaluation is recommended for any clinical rotation that extends for at least 6 days. If the rotation is fewer than 6 days, a mid-term evaluation is difficult to adequately complete. However, an informal meeting between you and the student may be prudent. The informal meeting might be as simple as a quick review of the evaluation form and your feedback regarding the student's performance to date. The meeting also may offer you the opportunity to discuss any early warning signs that you have observed in the student's performance.

CLINICAL OBJECTIVES

Assessing student performance at the clinical site can be a formidable task. The nursing instructor is not afforded the luxury of objective testing to measure student success. There is no fill-in-the-blank means of gauging the student's knowledge and safety on the floor, nor is there a multiple-choice test that can measure clinical effectiveness. Rather, the clinical teacher must base his or her judgment on direct observation within the context of written clinical objectives whose lack of precision can make them challenging to interpret. Examples of clinical objectives include the following:

- Demonstrates ability to meet the psychological needs of the critically ill client.
- Interprets own verbal and nonverbal communications accurately.
- Demonstrates appropriate interactions with all patients.

Different nursing instructors can interpret these objectives in various ways. How does a novice clinical instructor decide what information to note for later use in evaluating student performance in terms of the program's objectives?

"RED FLAG" WARNINGS

There is another aspect to becoming an astute clinical instructor. This involves awareness of the more common "red flags" that students may wave during their clinical rotation—signals that warrant an instructor's observation, concern, consultation, and action plan.

Here are some examples of "warning signs":

- **Hedging:** Students who arrive unprepared sometimes will try to answer your questions by hesitantly bringing up many unrelated facts. An example of "hedging" is when the instructor asks the student to explain why the client has intermittent compression devices on his legs after surgery. The student replies that it is for postop prevention of complications, but cannot specifically verbalize or describe the relevant complications that occur after surgery, nor can the student elaborate on nursing actions that prevent surgical complications. The student may offer other irrelevant details about the use of compression devices for orthopedic patients and the types of compression devices in the market. However the student does not provide a direct answer to your question. If the student does not know the specifics of why a nursing measure is taken, the student cannot evaluate the effectiveness of the measure.
- **Late submission of assignments:** Students are given a timetable for completing their assignments such as care plans, journals, and other assigned work. Students who submit their work late (on more than one occasion) may be having difficulty. It is possible that they have time

constraints related to employment and may be working too many hours to complete their school work in a timely manner. They may not be conscious of the need for timeliness in a field where it is necessary to be on time with nursing care. Late assignment submissions often have a cause that you as the instructor should investigate. Do not just think that you are helping the student by "letting it go." The vital importance that the timely completion of tasks plays in the care of the patient must be instilled at the outset.

- **Late arrival at the clinical site:** Nursing care is an ongoing process in which the arriving nurse continues the flow of care rendered by her predecessor from the preceding shift. Lateness can greatly compromise this continuity. Students must clearly understand that being late for the clinical is much more serious than being late for class. Unless the lateness is an unavoidable and isolated instance, such as a car accident, failure to appear at the designated hour is a very disconcerting sign. Do they really appreciate the tremendous responsibilities that accompany this profession? Are other parts of their lives interfering with their education? Whatever the cause, it is the clinical instructor's task to address the situation with the student, review consequences for any continued lateness, and evaluate the student's ability to continue meeting the objectives of the course and the clinical instructor's expectations.

- **Performing skills without supervision:** Chapter 4 provided information about the orientation day for the clinical instructor and new students. It was stated that upon arrival to a new hospital and unit, the rules and requirements of the host facility and school, and the instructor's expectations should be provided in writing and reviewed. Noted in this review would be the instruction that "no nursing skill should be performed or medication given by the student without supervision." The instructor should clearly state who can provide such supervision. Will it always be you, or are there circumstances when the professional nurse in your host facility is permitted to supervise the student? Some instructors require that students sign a statement at orientation day that they understand these requirements. Incorporate this prudent practice in your own clinical oversight, because a student who performs a task or skill without the appropriate supervision can cause a serious and potentially deadly error. Should a breach of the supervision rule occur, it is paramount that you act immediately! Have a conference with the student that day, if possible right after the incident. You usually need to report this error to the unit floor manager and your contact person or coordinator at the school of nursing. Follow the school's policies in this regard (see Chapter 2) and also be aware of its "safe practice" criteria (see Chapter 17).

• **Chronic personal crises:** Every instructor knows that "life happens." Anyone can have a bad day or perform in a manner that is not optimal. At the same time, be aware of the student who continually offers excuses for less than stellar clinical performance. For example, all students may be advised by the instructor to visit their nursing lab before the start of the clinical practicum in order to review certain procedures, such as insulin injections or administering medications through a feeding tube. If you notice that a particular student clearly does not know which step to take first to perform this required skill, obviously the student's preparation was not adequate. The student may offer reasons for poor performance, ranging from physical illness to emotional heartbreak. At first, many instructors will extend the benefit of the doubt and walk the student through the procedure. This forgiving approach, however, should include advising the student that the lack of preparation indicates that more review time is warranted with the lab coordinator and should be accompanied by appropriate documentation in the anecdotal notes. However, if you observe the same lack of preparation in the same student a second time, you have received a "warning sign."

TAKING ACTION ON WARNING SIGNS

What should the clinical instructor do about these warning signs? If you are relatively new to the field of clinical instruction, discuss these observations with a more experienced colleague. Clinical instructors develop their own methodologies for working with students. Courtesy would indicate that you notify the lab instructor in advance as to what you expect from the lab time. You may then send the student to the nursing lab with a written instruction of what specifically occurred during the clinical time. You may request a written note or email notification from the lab instructor confirming that the student did indeed complete the requested lab time. If enough warning signs accrue, the student may be in jeopardy of failing the clinical course. Familiarize yourself with the performance evaluation form and follow some of the suggestions in documenting unsafe practice in Chapters 9 and 17.

IMPORTANCE OF INTUITION

As you become a more experienced clinical instructor, you will rely more on your intuition. A student will impress you with some of his or her interactions with patients, and you will realize that you need not observe that student as keenly as others. These days, clinical instructors have a clinical group assignment with 6 to 10 students. With as many as 10 students, you need to develop a sense for determining which students need close scrutiny for patient safety and which are more competent in their skills.

Trust your instincts. You developed these similar instincts as a staff or primary nurse when you "just had a feeling" that the client was not doing well, and you spent additional time with that patient. It will be the same with student nurses. In time, your own instincts will alert you to the students who have a greater potential of possibly causing injury to the clients in their care.

FAST FACTS in a NUTSHELL

- Be alert for warning signs in students' performance.
- If you observe a warning sign, document it and seek advice when needed.
- Trust your instincts concerning "problem students."

11

Graded Clinical Versus Pass/Fail Evaluations

The time constraint inherent in clinical teaching has been acknowledged in this book. This is what makes the job of clinical instructors a bit more challenging than what is typically faced elsewhere in academia. However, because the profession of nursing is seen as a practice discipline at its core, students must be evaluated according to how they practice and, therefore, "perform." Clinical students can be graded with pass/ fail, satisfactory/unsatisfactory, letter/number grade, or a combination of these systems. Lastly, a brief word is offered about student evaluations of nursing instructors—how to learn from them and not be devastated by student criticism.

In this chapter, you will learn:

1. How each grading system works
2. The advantages and disadvantages of each system
3. Evaluation of the instructor by students

GRADING STUDENTS

In clinical teaching, the evaluation is the most difficult and emotionally charged responsibility (Scanlan, Care, & Gressler, 2001). Clinical instructors must deal with degrees of subjectivity in evaluating another person's performance, as well as with the fact that they do not have much time to spend with, let alone evaluate, students!

Challenges in Evaluating Students

Clinical instructors are consistently faced with several challenges in evaluating student performance. In some programs, an entire clinical rotation may last only 2 weeks. Moreover, the instructor is responsible for not just one student, but a group of students! For example, in a generic nursing program, the clinical instructor may be responsible for written evaluations and grades for as many as 10 students after a 7-week medical-surgical rotation.

Remember that often in nursing courses, there will be a separate classroom grade and a separate clinical grade for one course. Usually the student must pass both segments of the course to progress to the next step in the nursing program. There are some students who are superior test takers and do well in classroom courses but this does not always mean that they will also do well in the clinical component of the course. Clinical nursing courses are the essential component of nursing education that allow each student to transfer and apply learned knowledge into real situations.

Knowledge of Course Objectives

Instructors observe and score a student's performance based on a set of critical criteria linked to the course objectives.

Therefore, it is imperative that clinical instructors familiarize themselves with the clinical course objectives, set time for mid-term and final clinical evaluation periods, and, most importantly, be familiar with the grading system.

Unanticipated Events

In addition, anticipated and unanticipated events can affect the valuable time instructors have with students. For most clinical rotations, the first day is usually the assigned hospital orientation day. Other days may be lost to university or nursing program events that students are required to attend or legal holidays on which classes are canceled. Unanticipated events, such as extreme weather conditions or school disasters, may result in school closure. All of these events affect the number of days instructors have for observing and evaluating student performance.

TYPES OF GRADING SYSTEMS

The grading system for clinical courses is primarily based on the student's achievement of certain course objectives. Clinical courses are usually offered on a pass/fail grading system or letter/number grading system. See Exhibit 11.1 for a commonly used grading system that could be found in any student handbook.

Pass/fail grades and satisfactory/unsatisfactory grades are similar and do not provide comparative gradations among passing students. A letter grade offers a finer evaluation of a student's performance. Grading is usually specific to the nursing program. Exhibit 11.2 is another example of a grading system that would be found in a clinical course.

Exhibit 11.1   Grading System

The grading system used for nursing courses is based on the student's achievement of the course objectives. The grading scale is as follows:

Theory Course:

Letter Grade	Percentage Grade	Quality Points
A	93–100	4.0
B	84–92	3.0
C	75–83	2.0
F	Below 75	0.0

Clinical Laboratory:

S = Satisfactory
U = Unsatisfactory

Satisfactory or Unsatisfactory

Clinical laboratory is graded as satisfactory or unsatisfactory. A final grade of satisfactory is required in the clinical component of a nursing course. If the student is not demonstrating a pattern of satisfactory clinical performance, the clinical instructor will meet with the student to formulate a plan for improvement. Students must achieve all clinical course objectives/competencies by the end of the course to receive a satisfactory grade. An unsatisfactory clinical grade at the end of the course results in course failure regardless of grades received on classroom assignments, tests, and examinations. The final course grade will be recorded as an F.

**Exhibit 11.2   NSG 3116 Advanced Adaptation
Course**

NSL 3116 Clinical Course
Laboratory Component Grading System The grading
system used for nursing clinical courses is based on
the student's achievement of the course objectives. The
grading scale is as follows:

Pass or Fail
Clinical laboratory is graded as pass or fail. This means
that you will not receive a letter grade for the course;
rather, you will receive a grade of "P" for satisfactory
work and "F" for unsatisfactory work. Pass grades are
included in total credits earned but pass/fail grades are
not included in the grade point average.

CLINICAL EVALUATION FORMS

Clinical evaluation forms reflect the specific behavioral objectives of that course. To assist students in meeting these objectives, specific clinical criteria are established and written
out clearly on the evaluation form. These clinical criteria are
presented to the students and discussed with them on the first
clinical day. The student's performance and the instructor's
observations are the key elements in the evaluation process.

Evaluations of clinical criteria are clearly highlighted in
the clinical evaluation tool and may be given orally to the student by the instructor during the evaluation time.

CLINICAL OBJECTIVE EXAMPLE

An example of a clinical objective is: *The student applies knowledge of medical-surgical nursing when providing patient care.*

An instructor using the pass/fail grading system would report a P (pass) or an F (fail) for this objective based on that student's performance in the setting. In a program using the letter/number grading system, the instructor would score the student based on the rating scale. The scale is usually a Likert-type scale ranging from 1 to 5. See the example in Chapter 8. The scale scores for each objective would then be tallied to give a final clinical score.

Now consider your own evaluations that you will receive from the students that you teach. Most schools provide a system for your clinical students to evaluate the instructor at the end of each clinical rotation. Be kind to yourself when reading these evaluations. Most of the time, you will be pleased by what the students have to say, but heed this word of caution. Anyone who teaches nursing students long enough will receive a negative rating or comment at some point. It may not be possible to properly do the job that you are being entrusted with and always get glowing student evaluations. Talk over any negative evaluation with a trusted colleague. If comments are unfair and you fear consequences from your superiors, make an appointment with the coordinator of the course and explain the possible motivation of the particular student or group that rated you poorly.

FAST FACTS in a NUTSHELL

- Each program defines its own clinical evaluation system.
- Clinical objectives are highlighted in the clinical evaluation tool.
- A 1 to 5 rating scale is commonly used in a letter/number clinical grading system.
- Do not overreact to a negative student evaluation of your own performance.

Communication at Clinical Conferences

12

Preconferences

Preconferences are preclinical meetings held at the start of the clinical day. The conference is led by the instructor and can provide teaching and learning opportunities. These occur because the clinical instructor has the opportunity to assess the student's preparation and assignment for the clinical day and to observe key aspects of the student's communication skills that are necessary to nursing practice. Communication competence is an essential nursing skill because of the daily interactions nurses have with patients and other health care providers. Proper preparation for the clinical day is also essential and is an evaluation objective for all levels of nursing students.

In this chapter, you will learn:

1. The value and proper use of preconference time
2. The role of the preconference in relation to the objectives of the nursing process. One scenario of a type of preconference will be highlighted

WHAT IS A PRECONFERENCE?

During the clinical rotations, the instructor will schedule conferences. These conferences are usually held before the start of a clinical day and are called preconferences. If scheduled at the end of the day, they are called postconferences. For the clinical faculty, these conferences are a teaching-learning strategy because they are expected to follow up on elements from the classroom lectures. They also use these conferences to plan learning opportunities for their students. Among nurse educators, this is referred to as "the application of theory into practice."

STUDENT GUIDANCE

Each clinical instructor should remember that no one else is giving these students direction about the specific clinical rotation. Instructors are responsible for providing all guidance and addressing all questions regarding all aspects of the clinical experience. Their job responsibilities include setting the rules and structuring the clinical day according to the objectives of the program. Although students should learn the majority of the rules and instructor expectations on orientation day, conferences with students during the rotation also provide opportunities to share expectations and reinforce clinical guidelines.

Daily Expectations

Students will become frustrated if they do not know what is expected of them each clinical day. Students should not be surprised about the rules and guidelines nor should they arrive at a hospital unit without adequate preparation from the instructor. What kind of "preparation" is the clinical instructor responsible for? The instructor must "prepare" the students for his or her expectations and what is expected of their performance. This requires clarifying the clinical objectives set forth by the nursing program, which are usually broad and unspecific in relation to the actual elements of patient care. Each student needs to know the specific elements of patient care for which he or she will be responsible and the general timeline of each clinical day. This can best be done during a preconference.

Patient Care Assignments

The students usually receive their patient care assignments at this time. Many instructors are allowing students more latitude in choosing their patients for the day. If you give clear directions about which type of patient is best for the student to meet the objectives, the student can play the major role in choosing his or her patients with guidance from you and the unit's nursing staff. Remember your job is to foster independence and some sense of self-efficacy for each student. Use every opportunity to do so. If he or she received their patient assignment before the preconference, the clinical instructor can review each student's plan of care during the preconference. In essence, the purposes of a preconference are to give faculty an opportunity to prepare the students for the clinical day, to review any work from the students, and to set the structure of the clinical day to avoid frustration for all parties. An example of a preconference scenario is provided in Exhibit 12.1.

Exhibit 12.1   Preconference Scenario

At orientation day, Jason, the clinical instructor, informed students that at the beginning of each clinical day, at 6:30 a.m. sharp, he will hold a preconference with the group in the cafeteria meeting room. The purpose is to give them the three learning goals for the clinical day, as well as to give each of them their patient care assignment. At one particular preconference, Jason shared the following goals for students to fulfill on that clinical day: (1) to complete an assessment of their patient; (2) to document that assessment; and (3) to understand the medication list for each patient. Students were given these goals orally and on a written handout from the instructor. In addition, one student, Nancy, received a client in room 550, a 10-year-old patient with cystic fibrosis. The clinical instructor then directed Nancy and all the students to review the disease and its medical and nursing management during the rest of the preconference time.

In some programs, clinical instructors are expected to visit the site in advance of the clinical day to review and select patients for students, so that students can receive patient care assignments before the clinical day. If this is the expectation of your nursing program, then the preconference format may be structured differently than the preceding scenario. The preconference time can then be used to evaluate the student's understanding of a patient's disease and medical management and to assess adequate student preparation for the clinical day. The preconference time can also be used as a teaching opportunity. The nursing instructor may highlight a certain class of medications, such as salicylates, and have the students discuss its interactions and side effects. In addition, student communication skills may also be observed and evaluated. The instructor can inform students that preconference time will begin with each student stating his or her patient's initials, the diagnosis, medical and nursing management, and nursing goals.

When students receive patient care assignments in advance of the clinical day, the expectations are a bit different. There are higher expectations at the preconference and postconference because the students have more resources and time to prepare for the clinical day. Thus, the manner in which patient care assignments are distributed plays a role in the structure of the preconference session. However, throughout the clinical rotation, clinical faculty use these preconference sessions as evaluation opportunities to assess the student's clinical day preparation and review his or her knowledge of the nursing process.

FAST FACTS in a NUTSHELL

- The structure of the clinical nursing preconference is determined by the timing of the patient assignments.
- For the clinical instructor, the preconference is a time for teaching and learning opportunities.
- The preconference can also be used to evaluate each student's preparation and assessment of his or her patient assignment.

13

Postconferences

Postconferences are held at the conclusion of a clinical day. Students are usually expected to present their patients at the postconference. This time allows the instructor to address any events that may have occurred during the clinical day.

In this chapter, you will learn:

1. The purpose of postconferences
2. An explanation of their importance to the overall learning objectives of the clinical course and the analysis of patient care

WHAT IS A POSTCONFERENCE?

Preconferences and postconferences are similar. They are both meeting times at which clinical issues are discussed and questions about clinical objectives are answered by the instructor. In addition, postconference time is also seen by many as the best time for students to "debrief" about the events during their day. Debriefing is defined as an information-sharing event that consists of a conversation between peers (Hanna & Romana, 2007). To differentiate between the two conference times, most clinical faculty will lead the preconference, but follow the students' lead at the postconference. The reason is primarily associated with the timing of the conference. The conclusion of a long clinical day provides a better opportunity for the instructor to ascertain students' understanding of their patients' care and to question students about their findings from the chart and their own patient assessment.

TEACHING OPPORTUNITIES

Clinical faculty can use postconferences as teaching and student-learning opportunities. As such, the clinical instructor can, for example, review lab values with the clinical group at one postconference session. Or the postconference can be used to link class theory with actual practice elements. For example, if the class topic is respiratory obstructive disorders, during postconference, the instructor can elaborate on the lab values associated with this class of disorders. Or the postconference can focus on respiratory acidosis and the role played by arterial blood gases. In general, most postconference times are focused-learning events about the nursing process, fundamental concepts, or any client education principles. For example, the clinical instructor may have students review the Internet resources available as resources for clients and their families. You may also find some clinical instructors giving a "mini-test" about certain nursing care principles they want enforced. Most clinical faculty will plan many learning activities for their students. Another such activity is student presentations.

Student Presentations

Students can be assigned a 10-minute presentation on a nursing topic appropriate to the objectives of the clinical rotation. These student presentations can also be viewed as a communication assignment. Another assigned learning activity can relate to research articles. Depending on the level of the undergraduate student, the clinical instructor can collect literature reviews or have students verbalize some aspects of a research article during a postconference. Like a preconference, postconferences can take up to 1 hour. Because of time limitations, however, clinical instructors must designate this assignment from the start and provide students with an assigned due date for each learning assignment. Wink (1995) presents many alternative strategies for instructors to try during conferences. Read her article for more ideas.

Understand Conference Limitations

Do not overwhelm the conference time by including too many teaching-learning opportunities. Always be true to your students and be in touch with their psychosocial well-being. At the end of a clinical day during which they have been continuously evaluated, they are mentally and physically exhausted. *Know their limits.* This important tip will keep you from being frustrated as you set your own expectations for the postconference.

SHARING STUDENT EXPERIENCES

One word of caution about these conferences. Although clinical instructors often use preconferences and postconferences as an evaluation opportunity, not all conferences should be seen as evaluation time. The effective clinical instructor will also hold conferences that are devoid of the evaluation "hat." These conferences allow students to share experiences and interact with the group without the stress of performance evaluation. Inform your students when they will be specifically evaluated. Allow for free sharing of experiences. Once you do that, your conferences will run smoothly and will meet your expectations. If you choose, you can use the first 10 minutes of a postconference to ask and discuss an open-ended question, such as "For those who gave medications today, how did you like the experience?"

Because many teaching and learning opportunities exist, the clinical instructor should be cautioned not to try too many at once. Remember that postconferences can be a productive time for teaching and learning, a time when students have an opportunity to address concerns or voice issues regarding their patient care or their performance. Students may also question something that happened during the course of a day. Addressing concerns and questioning an event that may have occurred are examples of debriefing.

Sample Scenario

Exhibit 13.1 provides an example of an appropriate event to discuss at a postconference. As this exhibit illustrates, the student's assessment findings and the actions by the primary nurse can be a key discussion point for the postconference. In this scenario, the student verbalized key aspects of her patient's condition with the clinical group and shared the events that unfolded during her care of the patient. Students in this clinical group had many questions regarding the patient's diet and whether this could have been a factor related to the hypoglycemia.

Exhibit 13.1 Postconference Discussion Point

An undergraduate student in a progressive care unit was caring for a female patient recovering from open heart surgery and the complications of pneumonia. The patient could not speak because of a tracheostomy tube and was breathing room air. This was the second day the student was assigned to this patient. Knowing the patient from the previous day, the student noticed that the patient seemed more lethargic and became diaphoretic as she was completing the noon vital signs. The clinical instructor observed the student as she reported her findings to the assigned primary nurse. The blood glucose was quickly checked and revealed that the patient was acutely hypoglycemic. The primary nurse then alerted the physician.

Lessons Learned From the Scenario

This example provides many good observation points about this particular student. The student was able to effectively verbalize the event and share her experience with the group. More importantly, the clinical instructor observed her keen assessment of the patient as well as her actions of critical thinking (rechecking vital signs) and then her appropriate reaction (verbalizing her assessment concerns to the primary nurse).

Clinical instructors will find that time to actually stop and teach is limited during the course of a clinical day. The day progresses so quickly that many key events come and go without time to "pause" to share a key aspect of care or highlight a particular intervention. The time to do this is at postconference. When there is something to be emphasized, an item to be taught, or an event to debrief, postconferences provide the time to share and discuss experiences.

FAST FACTS in a NUTSHELL

- Postconference time should not be directed by the instructor. Rather, it is a time to debrief about the aspects of the day.
- Have postconferences without wearing the evaluation hat.
- Postconferences can be used as teaching and learning opportunities.

The Art of Making a Clinical Assignment

14

Unplanned Events

As any nurse or professional will tell you, the world of health care is filled with unexpected or unanticipated moments. In fact, aside from the nursing process itself, there is nothing "routine" in health and illness. Relay this fact to your students who are expecting to find the same patient in the same condition every day. Anticipating unplanned events, such as low census, acute changes in a patient's condition, resident outings, or client discharges, is key when developing an assignment that will provide the best learning experience for the student.

In this chapter, you will learn:

1. How to anticipate or plan in advance for changes in a student's clinical assignment
2. How to develop a "toolbox" of potential alternate assignments that will save time when unplanned events occur

PLANNING ASSIGNMENTS

It is sometimes impossible to predict the census or patient composition of the clinical unit to which your students have been assigned during their rotation. It may also be difficult to predict which clients will be available for your students to interact with at a retirement facility, day-care setting, or school. How can you, as the clinical instructor, plan an assignment for your charges and also ensure that your students are meeting their learning objectives for the clinical course?

First, you have to create a student nurse clinical assignment. Think of all of the potential clinical placements in which today's student nurses may find themselves. Students are at nursery schools, senior centers, maternity units, and community settings, to name a few. Thus, the development of a solid clinical assignment encompasses the clients in the clinical setting as well as awareness of the knowledge level and familiarity with nursing practice of the current groups of students in your practicum. This can be the most challenging task faced by all clinical instructors, especially during the first few weeks of the clinical rotation when you are just starting to distinguish each student and to begin assessing "high" versus the "not-so-high" fliers. Listed below are some standard guidelines that clinical instructors can use in all settings.

GUIDELINES FOR CLINICAL ASSIGNMENTS

- **Be familiar with the student evaluation tool,** which will list the clinical objectives.
- **Use this tool as your "roadmap"** for developing assignments.
- **Develop a relationship with the nursing staff** at your facility so its members can assist you.

- **Accept the nursing staff's hints and suggestions.** Their input is invaluable. For example, a staff nurse may tell you, "That patient is not good for a student." *Heed their advice.* They know. They will know what client has an anxious family who would be hesitant to allow a student nurse to care for their relative. They will also know the client who may be too threatening for a novice student.
- **Arrive a few hours before your students.** Arriving earlier will help you organize the clinical student assignment and provide time to talk to the staff and review the charts.
- **Inquire at the nursing report** (i.e., transfer of information about residents/clients from the current shift to the oncoming shift) about clients who would appreciate a student and learn those clients' schedules for that day. Will the clients be off of the unit most of the day for tests? Are they in too much pain to talk with the students on a day when a primary objective is oral communication?
- **Avoid writing down all of the patient data.** It is not your role to communicate this detailed level of information to the student. Part of the learning experience—and an essential component of your evaluation of each student—will be the student's understanding of what information is essential and where to locate that information. See Appendix C for a sample of a tool that can be shared with students electronically via an email message or can be posted in an online classroom environment commonly found in most nursing programs. Ensure that patient confidentiality is maintained when communicating via email. This means that no patient name is allowed. Room numbers or just initials may be used.
- **Be cognizant of each student's strengths and weaknesses.** For example, a student who has some initial self-confidence issues may not be the one to take on the cantankerous older adult patient who will "order" her

around all day. Students who are able to handle more difficult clients may appropriately receive a higher grade or be given a more positive evaluation, than other students.

- **Be flexible.** The most detailed and well-prepared assignment may fall apart when clients are not available on the scheduled day or are unable to accept a student for some reason. A sense of humor will serve you well on these days.

UNPLANNED EVENTS

Here is the irony. Although most learning opportunities are planned in a clinical rotation, in acute care settings where illness, death, and various human experiences are the reality, you can be sure that "unplanned" events will likely occur. Try to have a "back-up" plan when creating a student assignment. This can be accomplished by carrying with you relevant clinical case studies to use if circumstances result in a student's inability to complete objectives on a given day. For example, the student may have planned to perform a psychosocial assessment on the assigned client, but that client has unexpectedly left for the day. The staff states that no other client is available, so the student and client have agreed to complete the assessment on the following day. This is an opportune time to give the student the case studies you are carrying, with the objective of reviewing and then presenting them to his or her peers at a postconference.

Another example of an unplanned event could be the student who is overwhelmed halfway into the shift. He or she shares some fear that the client's needs will not be met that day during the scheduled time with the client. You can always assign a second student to provide assistance. Often, that second student will be the one who is able to complete most of the responsibilities more quickly than the other. Working together teaches students that helping one another is essential to the practice of nursing. Often, students learn best from a peer. The peer can teach the slower student some "tricks of the trade" in a nonthreatening manner that is beneficial to all. As you detect differences in the students' abilities, capture your observations in the anecdotal notes, as mentioned in Chapter 9.

ALTERNATIVE ASSIGNMENTS

Lastly, develop a list of alternative assignments that can be employed with your students when needed. Chapter 15 will describe in detail what is meant by "alternative assignments."

FAST FACTS in a NUTSHELL

- Preparation for student assignments will often prove beneficial.
- Unplanned events will occur despite your best plans.
- Flexibility and a positive relationship with the staff at your facility will assist you in adapting a student assignment.

15

Alternative Assignments

All levels of students (from first to final year) will benefit from assignments "outside" of the specified clinical rotation. Supplemental experience in a department other than the assigned one enhances the educational value of the clinical site. This alternative assignment can occur in the community or pediatric, maternity, psychiatric, or medical-surgical rotations of a student's clinical experience. As noted in Chapter 14, it is helpful to have a plan for the "unplanned events" that inevitably occur on many clinical days. This chapter presents samples of alternative assignments based on the particular clinical rotations. They are accompanied by tips on methods for coordinating and cultivating these alternative assignments to benefit all parties, but especially the students.

In this chapter, you will learn:

1. The value of providing alternative assignments for your students
2. Sample alternative assignments for many different clinical rotations that instructors can use immediately in their current work

MEETING PROGRAM OBJECTIVES

In all types of nursing programs—associate, diploma, or baccalaureate—the "guiding light" of your clinical rotations are the clinical objectives specified on the evaluation tool. Some schools use generic objectives that can be applied to multiple locations, such as maternity, pediatric, or psychiatric nursing settings. Other schools may have different objectives for each specific rotation. No matter what the evaluation tool, the instructors must follow these objectives and plan opportunities for all students to meet each program objective. This is often challenging. Remember that you may have up to 10 students in your rotation, and each must be given an equal opportunity to meet the required objectives.

ALTERNATIVE ASSIGNMENTS

For this reason, it is prudent to develop "alternative assignments" for each clinical rotation. These alternative assignments serve many purposes. They offer a chance to carry the stated purpose and knowledge of this rotation to a different location, where the student can often interact with different staff personnel. Another purpose of these alternative assignments is to create a more manageable number of students for you to evaluate and supervise on any given day. For example, an instructor has 10 students on an acute pediatric hospital unit to supervise. Several of these students need to administer medications, and all need to complete comprehensive patient care. This is a formidable task for any instructor. If two or three alternative assignments were created that met some of the clinical objectives of this pediatric rotation, then the instructor would have only 7 nursing students on the acute care floor instead of 10.

Appropriate Assignments

An important caveat to these alternative assignments is that they need to facilitate the students' attempts to meet their clinical objectives and that the level coordinator needs to agree with your assessment of this alternative as safe and beneficial. An example of how these assignments can be abused or deemed inappropriate is shown in Exhibit 15.1.

Exhibit 15.1   Inappropriate Alternative Assignment

Megan, a new nursing clinical instructor, supervised nine students for a 4-day rotation through an acute psychiatric unit. At an orientation session, the level or course coordinator communicated the clinical objectives to this instructor. The school has used this site for many years, and the school and unit nurses had a good working relationship.

Megan decided unilaterally that nine students were too many to supervise at one site. Without asking the level or course coordinator, she asked the facility's emergency department (ED) if she could send two students to the ED on each of the three clinical days and three students on a fourth day. All would therefore have the same opportunity.

The students reported this practice to the coordinator. The students were concerned about missing the needed opportunity to care for patients and meet their assigned objectives with them on an acute psychiatric unit. Because this was only a 4-day rotation, their concern was well-founded. They all enjoyed the ED

(continued)

Exhibit 15.1   *(continued)*

experience but knew that they were not meeting their primary objectives.

The level or course coordinator called the new instructor; they met privately to review the course and clinical objectives. The course coordinator also reminded the clinical instructor to keep all students on the acute psychiatric unit as prescribed by the nursing curriculum. Megan was asked why she had assigned these students to an alternative placement like the ED during their brief psychiatric rotation. She responded that she thought students would have an opportunity to observe clients who came to the ED when in acute psychiatric crisis. Although there was a possibility that this could occur, it was unlikely. Moreover, Megan is now aware that she is required to check with the level or course coordinator before any alternative assignment was created.

With the above example in mind, remember that although alternative assignments can and often are beneficial, they must adhere to the clinical objectives of the rotation and must receive the level coordinator's approval. Table 15.1 illustrates some possible alternative assignments for students in different rotations. Each instructor needs to modify these suggestions to his or her school's specifications and requirements.

Clinical Rotation Assignments

TABLE 15.1 Samples of Possible Alternative Assignments

Clinical Rotation	Alternative Assignment
Acute hospital pediatric floor	Day with a pediatric nurse practitioner
Maternity rotation in hospital	Visit to a free-standing birth center
Acute psychiatric rotation	Visit to an outpatient community mental health center
Medical-surgical floor	Day in the critical care unit
Community health	Day at a migrant farm location

These are only a few of the creative and valuable alternative assignments that you can have in your repertoire. You must also give students clear instructions with each alternative assignment. For example, the student who spends the day with the pediatric nurse practitioner during his or her pediatric rotation must have a written format with objectives and requirements for that day.

Importance of Feedback

A written assignment describing how the above objectives were or were not fulfilled during that student's day may be required. It is also advisable to get feedback from the nurse practitioner about the student's performance. Exhibit 15.2 provides an example of instructions for an alternative assignment.

Exhibit 15.2 Assignments for Clinical Rotations

During your experience with the pediatric nurse practitioner, you will be concentrating on Objectives 1, 2, and 3 of your evaluation tool, which read:

1. Observe the role of each nurse in his or her relationship with ill children and in performing nursing responsibilities.
2. Familiarize yourself with the Nurse Practice Act and observe the nurse's extended role as a practitioner.
3. Assess the nursing process used with each pediatric client during your experience.

Some examples of negative feedback would be:
   "The student just sat in the corner of the office and read through journals."
   "I attempted to engage the student and often pointed out different assessment findings, but the student just looked, said little, and returned to a corner seat."

This feedback is invaluable. These data could alert you to one of the early warning signals mentioned in Chapter 10. What is interfering with a student's ability to learn? Is it lack of motivation? Lack of sleep? Something is amiss, and it is now your opportunity to address the problem and try to correct it.

It is important that students do not view an alternative assignment as a "day off." Convey this information by carefully orienting students to the goals and written assignment for the day. Let the student know that you will talk to the nurses at the alternative assignment setting and receive feedback.

Prepare the Clinical Setting

As the clinical instructor, it is important to "scope" out the alternative assignment site and experience it for yourself before assigning a student. Verify that the nursing staff is willing to teach and have a student "shadow" them for the day. Be clear with the staff and management about the specifics of the student's assignment. For example, if the student is spending the day with the pediatric nurse practitioner, make sure that the student does not assess or document or perform any procedure while at the site. The student would probably not be covered for any liability if in a different locale or part of the clinical rotation. Stress that this is an observation experience only and be very clear with your students about the parameters of their responsibilities on that day.

Individualizing Student Assignments

Although there are general rules or guidelines for each chapter of this book as they pertain to student education, each student's clinical experience needs to be individualized. For example, perhaps a student is struggling on the assigned unit. The student may have made a medication error or missed an important client assessment. Under these circumstances, carefully consider the appropriateness of giving the student an alternative assignment. You may not be able to observe this student at that assignment, and the student may need more time to meet the objectives of your specific unit. If this is true, do not send this student to the alternative assignment. Inform the student why this is occurring. Explain that you need more intensive time to observe his or her performance and that he or she needs more opportunity to master the objectives of this specific clinical site. Informing your level coordinator is again a wise step in case the student complains about this change.

It is also imperative that instructors document the "why" and "how" of these decisions. Refer to Chapter 9 on how to document the performance of a student who is at risk of failing.

FAST FACTS in a NUTSHELL

- Alternative assignments serve many practical purposes.
- These assignments must be meaningful and approved.
- Specific clinical objectives must be established for each alternative assignment, with written and oral feedback from the student.

PART

VII

Competencies Not Met

16

Punctuality and Absences

Each clinical course runs for a specific number of clinical hours and days, so that competencies are maintained. Students are required to arrive on time and be present each and every clinical day. Absences and tardiness affect the performance of students and must be monitored closely by the clinical instructor.

In this chapter, you will learn:

1. The impact of absences and lateness on meeting clinical objectives
2. A summary of the set policies concerning clinical absences and tardiness

BASIC COMPETENCIES IN THE CLINICAL SETTING

The student is assigned functions and responsibilities that are necessary to pass each clinical rotation. These rotations take place in various work environments, such as public health and community agencies, homes, schools, clinics, hospitals, and nursing homes. General responsibilities and assigned functions encompass those required for nursing practice and may include assessing a patient, planning and delivering care, performing acute care interventions, providing direct care safely, teaching patients and their family members, and teaching community residents about health and illness. Students must also be competent in reviewing the patient's medical condition, summarizing the patient's chart, assessing health and illness, carrying out the physician's orders, and communicating with all parties. These are basic competencies for students in clinical settings.

To evaluate a student's performance, a certain number of days and a set number of hours are for the clinical instructor's review. Even then, clinical instructors often find that the clinical rotation time is too short. Therefore, *instructors frown on student absences or tardine*ss because it further minimizes the time available for student evaluation. Instructors are responsible for enforcing all policies pertaining to this conduct.

ABSENCES

This is not to say that clinical educators want students who are ill to care for patients. But *the student is responsible for informing the instructor* of an illness the night before or on the day of the clinical experience.

For a prolonged and unexpected student absence, the routine procedure is for the assigned faculty to discuss the situation and designate a plan of action for that student. Each case needs individual attention by the designated faculty. Clinical instructors are never alone in making these decisions.

The nursing program has a set policy regarding absences that is strictly enforced. Clinical instructors are told to seek the assistance of the course coordinator regarding habitual policy violators. Most nursing programs have set mechanisms and procedures that clearly identify what students have to do in the event of a clinical absence, whether excused (documentation of illness from a health care provider) or unexcused (no documentation or evidence supporting the absence).

Make-Up Assignments

For minor illnesses, a "make-up assignment" or "make-up clinical time" is the routine plan. Some nursing programs allow the student to make up the clinical experience on another day either with the regular clinical instructor or another instructor. Students are required to pay "out of pocket" for this make-up time (based on a set fee structure). Other programs routinely prefer to provide "make-up work" for the student. Examples of such work can be a research article critique, a literature review presentation, or the completion of several case studies from a workbook. Make-up work should be collected within a week of the absence. It is wise to check with the program's course coordinator for other examples of acceptable make-up work. At this time, there is no evidence to support using simulated learning in a lab to replace actual time spent with clients and patients in a clinical practicum experience. Moreover, each nursing program usually has a designated lab area designed for self-directed student learning. Other worthwhile assignments may be extracted from this environment.

Clinical instructors should designate make-up work that can assist the students in meeting the required clinical objectives. However, *constant or prolonged absences are a detriment to the student's overall progress* and prevent successful achievement of the objectives. This leads to a poor clinical grade and clinical/academic failure. *Make sure you track student absences.* It is recommended that at the second absence, the instructor contacts the program's coordinator for feedback on managing this issue. The program may already have a procedure in place for such issues.

If you need to devise make-up work, it is wise to have students complete assignments related to the clinical practicum or related to the nursing theory (didactic) course in which they are currently enrolled. Exhibits 16.1 and 16.2 offer examples of make-up assignments that you can apply to your student groups.

Exhibit 16.1   Written Make-Up Assignments
for Clinical Absence

A.   The instructor will assign a literature review on a medical-surgical nursing topic. The paper will be graded on the content and the format required for a literature review.

   The literature review will include a title page and a reference page (current). It will be a minimum of six pages, with the format and margins as required by the latest edition of the *Publication Manual of the American Psychological Association* guidelines.

   Due date: 10 days from absence.

B.   The instructor will assign three case studies to be completed by the following Thursday.

Exhibit 16.2   Oral Make-Up Assignments for Clinical Absence

Guidelines for an Ethical–Legal Presentation
1. Select an ethical or legal topic from the pediatric or medical-surgical nursing specialties as the basis for a discussion or debate
2. Review the literature and provide a 5-minute presentation (including a written outline to be shared with the group) using one of the following techniques:
    • Focus on a recent debate issue
    • Highlight a recent news item on the issue
    • Present the research problem and identify a question
    • Present a case study from your experience
    • Summarize the literature
3. Lead a 5-minute discussion on this topic
4. Bonus points: Any creativity brought to the presentation

TARDINESS

As with absences, the *clinical instructor should monitor student tardiness from the first day* of the clinical experience. Students can be tardy for numerous reasons, such as car problems and road conditions. However, the student should not offer these excuses to explain a pattern of tardiness. If a student arrives late every Tuesday morning, then the student has a responsibility problem and should be evaluated accordingly.

Each time a student is tardy, the instructor should be informed as early as possible. As soon as the student arrives, he or she must immediately seek the clinical instructor for a briefing on what was missed. The clinical instructor can usually assign a late-arriving student with another student or to shadow a staff member (with the staff's permission). Such adjustments depend on the location of the clinical experience, as student responsibilities and duties vary by setting. If a student has a pattern of lateness, that student will probably not meet some of the clinical objectives. This will affect the student's overall clinical grade. It is recommended that clinical instructors inform the faculty coordinator to discuss any absent or tardy student as soon as possible.

FAST FACTS in a NUTSHELL

- Nursing programs value punctuality.
- Clinical absences require make-up work.
- Nursing programs have strict policies regarding absences and tardiness.

17

Unsafe Practice

Standards of care for nursing professionals emphasize safe and competent practice. As a result, most programs have clearly defined policies regarding safe and unsafe practice. There is zero tolerance for any unsafe practice.

In this chapter, you will learn:

1. A detailed example of an unsafe practice event
2. The requirements for the instructor who encounters a similar event

SAFE PRACTICE

Nursing programs have a moral and ethical responsibility to prepare graduates who will be competent and safe caregivers. This obligation is clearly spelled out by the American Nurses Association (ANA). In some programs, safe practice is documented as adequate knowledge of the nursing process and safe performance of skills, such as patient assessment and medication administration. In other programs, safe practice involves behaviors that uphold the ANA Code of Ethics. Clinical educators must be aware that the concept of "safe or unsafe practice" is not commonly defined by all nursing programs. The clinical instructor is encouraged to seek this definition (if applicable) in the student handbook or ask the level or course coordinator if there is a policy and definition.

ANA Code

The ANA's Code of Ethics (2001) requires that "the nurse acts to safeguard the client and public when healthcare and safety are affected by the incompetent, unethical, or illegal practice of any person." Both students and faculty have this ethical duty. Students should be well aware of the rules and standards before beginning each rotation.

What Is an Unsafe Event?

As discussed earlier, it is incumbent on clinical instructors to understand all policies and procedures for evaluating students. Exhibit 17.1 is an example of an unsafe event involving student Mary Pat and a clinical instructor. For some, it may be surprising that this is classified as an unsafe event, as it did not cause direct "harm," or is not classified as a "medication error." These are the most commonly thought of unsafe practice events.

However, in this example, the student not only acted beyond her authorized role, she did not follow the nursing process by completing a patient assessment before any intervention. The clinical instructor met with the student the next day and had the student read the written report of the day's event. The student understood she was being cited for unsafe practice and that she had not properly followed the nursing process. The student confirmed her understanding by signing the bottom of the event report sheet.

Exhibit 17.1   Unsafe Practice Event

Clinical instructor, Cindy, was at the opposite end of the hall when she saw her student, Mary Pat, looking quite stressed. The clinical instructor quickly made her way into the room of Mary Pat's patient. She observed Mary Pat's apprehensiveness and the fact that the patient's intravenous (IV) bag was empty. Mary Pat's patient had been bathed and was reading the paper on a chair next to her bed. Everything looked neatly organized, but there was a ringing noise coming from the IV pump. It seemed that the IV bag and IV line were empty. Cindy quickly turned off the IV pump, while also clamping the IV bag. Cindy also observed that the IV tubing was looped incorrectly into the IV pump, as a key filter was not attached. She asked Mary Pat how long the IV had been ringing, and Mary Pat answered, "only a few minutes." Mary Pat shared that the patient asked to be bathed and then helped into the chair. Cindy informed Mary Pat that the pump was ringing because the bag and tubing had air in them. She also added, "Did someone come in and disconnect the tubing from the pump?" Mary Pat acknowledged that she had to disconnect the bag and tubing so that she could change the gown

(continued)

Exhibit 17.1 *(continued)*

after the bath. Cindy picked up the nurse's assessment flow sheet and asked Mary Pat to join her in the hallway. Once in the hallway she guided Mary Pat into the clean utility room, "Do you know what was running in the IV bag?" Mary Pat looked hesitant and did not quickly offer an answer but started looking for her handwritten notes from that morning's report. She answered, "Normal saline with potassium?" Cindy commented to Mary Pat, "That bag has been infusing with heparin, which you did not document on the morning report. Two weeks ago, you also had a patient with a heparin infusion. We assessed and documented that case together. More important, the tubing was not attached to the pump correctly, so this patient may have received more heparin than she should have. Do you understand that this is a major event? We will have to report this to the primary nurse and the physician. We will also have to fill out an event report and follow the policy accordingly. But, first, let us find the primary nurse to see what he wants us to do next."

That afternoon, after the postconference, Cindy told Mary Pat to meet her in her office the next day to discuss the seriousness of the morning's event. She told Mary Pat that she saw the event as an "unsafe practice" and would need to share a written report of the situation and follow the policy on unsafe practice as documented in the student handbook. She asked Mary Pat if she had any questions regarding her comments. Mary Pat said "No," but then she quickly added, "I had taken the IV lines off the pump before . . . when I worked as a patient care technician. I sometimes had to get patients ready for their tests so I detached them from the pumps. The staff nurses have seen me do this many times."

(continued)

Exhibit 17.1 *(continued)*

The instructor explained to Mary Pat that even though she had worked with IVs as a patient care technician, she was functioning now only as a student—and not as a technician. Therefore, she was not allowed to disconnect IV lines during her clinical rotation without the supervision of the clinical instructor. The clinical instructor also stressed that the role of the student was discussed extensively on orientation day and she also showed Mary Pat that it was explicitly stated in writing in the clinical handouts the students received.

The clinical instructor then followed the policy at this particular nursing program by discussing the incident with the level or course coordinator. At faculty meetings, unsafe practice events are discussed. This raises faculty awareness and draws attention to students who have "patterns" of unsafe practice events in their records. All instructors should have a thorough understanding of the nursing program's policy on unsafe practice (if any). There should not be any ambiguity in the clinical setting regarding the clinical instructor's role in the event of such situations.

ASSESSING SAFE PRACTICE

Because the *primary goal of nursing education is to train safe and competent nurses* who are accountable for their actions, clinical educators have a legal, ethical, and professional responsibility to assess students for safe practice (Smith, McKoy, & Richardson, 2001). In some cases, clinical educators may be reluctant to enforce this unsafe practice policy because of unclear direction by their nursing programs. They simply may not have had previous experience in enforcing this policy, or they may not be sure that their student evaluation will be upheld and supported by program officials.

Failing a Student for Unsafe Practice

In addition, instructors may face challenges from failing students. Students will usually challenge upsetting academic decisions in a process that some colleges and universities call "grievance." The student's family may also become involved. All of these psychosocial aspects are challenging to the clinical instructor. It is generally more work and aggravation to fail a clinical student than to simply let the student pass. However, the ethical and legal responsibilities remain. Clinical educators are hired to assess and assist their students. Nursing programs are designed to produce students who can satisfactorily and safely perform skills.

Examples of Unsafe Practice

Instructors should be alerted to examples of unsafe practice events. Additional unsafe events include:

1. **The student has not prepared for assigned tasks.** The student was given an assignment to review all aspects of patient medications before administering them, but arrives on the clinical day without having looked up or prepared any of the medications.
2. **A student has not reported abnormal vital signs to the staff nurse or clinical instructor.** An adult patient had a temperature of 102°F in a postprocedure setting, but the student did not report this abnormal vital sign value.
3. **A student has given medications without the presence of the clinical instructor.** Students must be made aware that they are practicing nursing tasks and duties under the license and guidance of the clinical instructor. This information is in the rules and guidelines they received on their orientation day. Not following these rules should mandate an unsafe practice report.

FAST FACTS in a NUTSHELL

- The clinical instructor must be aware of the ANA Code of Ethics.
- Each nursing program has its own definition of safe and unsafe practices.

18

What Your Students Will Expect of You

Now that you are prepared to enter the world of a clinical nursing instructor, it will be important to focus on what your students will expect of you. You have clearly informed them, on their orientation day, about all of your expectations as well as those of the nursing school. Now it is time to think about their expectations of you.

In this chapter, you will learn:

1. The four important attributes or traits that students expect in a clinical nursing instructor
2. The ABCs of developing a successful and professional relationship with your students
3. The importance of developing a self-care philosophy and practice

STUDENT EXPECTATIONS OF INSTRUCTORS

You have prepared well for your new role as a clinical nursing instructor. You have read this book and used its "blueprints" to prepare for your orientation day, student evaluations, and unit orientation.

You know what you expect of yourself, but what do your students expect of you? Although they may never verbalize their expectations, students require several vital qualities in their instructor. That is why successful clinical nursing instructors remember to bring their CAP to clinical each day. This CAP is not the iconic headpiece worn by nurses in the past, but rather a mnemonic that captures the essential traits you must always exhibit to your charges:

C   consistency
A   approachability
P   proficiency

CONSISTENCY

Nursing students are usually quite anxious on their first clinical day of each rotation. There often are rumors that upper classmates have circulated about the clinical instructor, the unit, and the workload of each rotation. The first day is often marked by shaking legs, nervous stares, and sweaty palms. This is not all bad. It is important for each student to appreciate the seriousness of the responsibility that he or she has at the clinical site, as well as the corresponding burden of responsibility borne by the clinical nursing instructor. In each circumstance, a facility's professional staff is allowing you and your students to enter their domain and care for their clients. The trust that the clients place in the facility is temporarily transferred to you.

The students must realize this and must trust you to help them navigate this unfamiliar territory. They trust you to provide adequate orientation; to establish safe limits and boundaries in terms of their roles; to ask them questions that pinpoint their areas of weakness; and to have a cohesive working relationship with the unit staff that will aid and benefit their education. Students must also be secure in their knowledge of who you are and what you expect. As such, you must exhibit consistency in your day-to-day oversight of their activities.

What does this mean? It means that you have to stick to your word and to what you have documented in handouts provided to students during orientation day or some time at the beginning of the rotation. If you say that you will email their assignments to them by 4 p.m., you must do so. It means that if you say that one journal is due each week and provide the guidelines for it, you stick to that expectation and format. You cannot change the expectations after the rotation begins. Consider the examples in Exhibit 18.1.

Exhibit 18.1   Consistency

Case 1

Kate is an instructor with one or two students who complain that the workload of a weekly journal assignment is too much with all of their other course responsibilities. They request that she reduce this assignment. However, most of the other students are having no difficulty completing the task and find the assignment helpful for their learning. Kate changes the assignment to resolve the complaint.

Case 2

Jerry is an instructor who tells his students on orientation day that he requires that they know the category, dose, and side effects of all of their medications. Then, on medication day, he goes further and asks them about the chemical composition, actions, and half-life of the medications.

Case Evaluation

In the first case, the instructor lowered her stated expectations, while in the second case, the instructor increased what he originally asked of his students. Both instructors lacked consistency and were ultimately unfair to their students. Vacillating expectations only serve to undermine student trust in the instructor.

Trustworthiness

Trustworthiness and consistency are intertwined. To be reliable as a nursing clinical instructor, students should often be able to predict your actions and reactions. For example, if they do not submit their journal to you on the appropriate day, they need to know from the outset that you will subtract 5 points from their grade unless they experienced a real emergency. Everyone, including the star student who is the nursing clinical genius and the struggling student who may be in jeopardy of failure, must know the policy. Consistency demands the same treatment for the same quality of work. *There can be no favoritism.*

Therefore, if you expect the students to be on the unit for clinical at 6:45 a.m., then you too are on the unit at that time. Although no clinical instructor is immune to the risk of a flat tire, a roadblock, a storm, or other situation that can delay arrival at the clinical site, these situations should be the exceedingly rare exception. Be where you are supposed to be, and on time!

Evaluation Policies

You also need to be consistent with your evaluation policies. If you say that the end of the clinical day is at 2 p.m., do not make an exception for a student who may have an appointment. For example, students may ask to leave early because they have a professional nursing job interview. Keep in mind, however, that clinical time is valuable and already limited, so you do not want to take time away from the experience. In addition, if other students see that you are inclined to grant exceptions, you can expect them to present you with other types of early-dismissal requests.

Consistency also means if you tell a student you will supervise her insertion of a urinary catheter in her patient's room in 15 minutes, you are in fact there to supervise her at the appointed time. If an emergency delays you, send a second student down to inform the first student as to why you are not there and make other arrangements. A student will become extremely frustrated if he or she is waiting for your arrival and you do not show. The client loses trust in the student, and the student will lose trust in you.

The trust your students place in you will be earned by the fairness and reliability that you consistently project.

APPROACHABILITY

Because students are highly anxious as they embark on a new clinical rotation, you must establish standards, guidelines, and rules. At the same time, however, you must remain approachable. What does this mean? Approachable means that you explain your rationale for your actions and ask for student feedback.

Approachable also means that you get to know each student's name and use his or her name and pronounce it correctly. Approachable means that you announce on the very first day that you understand that each student is an individual with different learning needs and different experiences. For example, some of your students may have worked as unlicensed assistive personnel or nursing technicians in health care facilities and have, therefore, learned many skills. Others may have been care providers in a different kind of facility. You must emphasize that you realize the differences and that all the objectives can be met by each student despite their varying degrees of exposure to working in a health care setting. State emphatically that you want students to tell you when they do not know something. The benefits of this policy are shown in Exhibit 18.2.

Exhibit 18.2 Approachability

During her psychiatric rotation, a senior student was responsible for taking the blood pressure of the clients on the unit. She seemed very upset by this assignment and explained to the instructor that on her job, she took blood pressure using a noninvasive automatic blood pressure cuff and had therefore forgotten how to take blood pressure manually. It was important for this senior nursing student to feel that the instructor was approachable in this situation. It allowed the instructor to review the student's technique and required the student to return to the nursing skills lab for practice.

Fairness

It is vital for students to feel that you are approachable as they deliver care to their clients. If the student makes an error or even thinks that he or she has made an error, the student will be concerned and anxious. At the same time, the student should feel that his or her concern and anxiety are not barriers to immediately coming to you with the problem.

Being approachable does not mean that you are a buddy or friend to your students. It means that they are aware that you are there to help them succeed. Your approachability will be demonstrated by your ability to remain reasonable and emotionally controlled when your assistance is needed concurrently in multiple places, when you are behind in your schedule, or when you are just not feeling up to par. Remaining approachable is paramount for the safety of the patients and the security of the students caring for them.

PROFICIENCY

As the instructor, you are the acknowledged expert. Your students watch your technique carefully and rely on your advice. The nursing staff depends on your expertise to ensure that no harm comes to their patients as a result of student inexperience. So what exactly is your level of expertise in a field whose breadth of information and practice seemingly evolves by the day? Unless you make a continued effort to keep your knowledge current, you cannot discharge your role effectively. See Exhibit 18.3 for an example of the importance of proficiency.

Exhibit 18.3 Proficiency

At the start of the fall semester, Rhonda brought her new class to the medical-surgical floor on which she had not worked for the past 4 years. The first day quickly turned into a nightmare, as Rhonda realized that the process of dispensing medications had become automated with optically scanned barcodes. Because of the security embedded in the new technology, she had no means of accessing the system and no idea how to use it once it was accessed. The students were not able to complete the fundamental chore of administering medications, and Rhonda's credibility suffered in the eyes of staff and students alike.

Case Evaluation

How can such an unfortunate situation be avoided? Start by subscribing to professional publications. These timely periodicals can offer valuable information on how research and technical innovation are affecting nursing care, often before these innovations are widely introduced into practice. It is also a good idea to keep in touch with the nurse manager, who can be a considerable asset in this regard. Innovations are usually introduced with sufficient lead time to allow for their incorporation into the daily routine. Just as the staff nurses get on-site training, so too should you. Since it may not be appropriate or feasible to participate in the training provided to the nursing staff, take the initiative to shadow a staff nurse for the day (with permission of course). This investment of time will pay dividends later, when all student eyes turn to you for instruction in a new skill.

Remember that you too were once a nursing student. The expectations you had of your instructors are likely no different from those that your students now have of you. They depend on you, and they need to trust you. You will earn their trust through consistency, approachability, and proficiency. Among your students you may very well have a future nursing instructor who will emulate the example you set today.

FAST FACTS in a NUTSHELL

- Your students have many expectations of you.
- Anticipate student expectations and strive to meet them.
- When you enter the clinical site, do not forget your CAP: consistency, approachability, and proficiency.

PART

VIII

The Growing Importance
of Reference Letters and Simulation

19

Letters of Reference

This chapter focuses on the growing importance that prospective employers place on letters of reference written by clinical nursing instructors. Address this topic with your students on orientation day to set their expectations in this regard appropriately. Before you do, consider these questions: What is your legal responsibility to provide these letters? What do nurse recruiters say about the value of reference letters? How can you write a meaningful and valuable letter in a specific time frame when you have so many other responsibilities? Sample letters of reference are provided in Appendix D.

In this chapter, you will learn:

1. The importance of establishing written guidelines for your students regarding your "rules" for letters of reference
2. How to navigate the scenario when a "not-so-high flier" requests you to write a reference
3. About online surveys from employers and agencies such as "skillsurvey .com" and what may be expected of you in completing these surveys

LETTERS OF REFERENCE

According to researchers from the RAND Corporation, Vanderbilt University, and Dartmouth College, the number of people ages 23 to 26 who became RNs increased by 62% from 2002 to 2009. There is one thing that most of these new RNs had in common—they needed at least one letter of reference from their nursing instructors in their pursuit of jobs.

As a clinical nursing instructor, just how valuable is your letter of reference for a particular student?

Perhaps this question is best answered by the employer. Rita Linus, nurse residency coordinator/nursing student facilitator for Main Line Health System in Pennsylvania, kindly offers the following insights for all clinical nursing instructors:

What are you looking for in letters of reference?

Clear descriptors of their performance—always.

It's great to see where they rank in the educator's experience estimation. If they say the job candidate is one of the best students they ever instructed or falls into the top 5% of students, this makes it pretty easy!

What have you seen in letters of references that would be a "turn-off"?

General, nondescriptive letters offer little value to a nurse recruiter.

How much weight do the letters of reference really have in the nursing job hire process?

In evaluating a nursing candidate, a letter of reference represents about 30% of the total application screening tool.

What might be a "red flag" to the employer in reviewing these letters?

Narrative form letters that just change student names and offer little or no insight as to the job applicant's performance are a red flag. Conversely, template evaluations for ranking student performance are nice because they are based on consistent criteria, and comments in addition to those measures are greatly appreciated.

Do you prefer receiving recommendations from clinical instructors or classroom instructors?

In the hiring process, letters of recommendation from clinical nursing instructors are requested.

What area of clinical instruction specialty do you find to be the most helpful?

That can vary. If they are applying for OB, it's nice to see an OB clinical recommendation. Just an aside … often we see recommendations from psych rotations and/or community study. These are value-added as well but if the applicant's interest is ICU, it doesn't provide us with as much clinical experience as a leadership rotation or tele/ICU experience.

Final words from Rita…

In our evaluation of their application, we look at leadership/ participation, volunteer activity, and professional organization membership, as well as current and past work experience (nursing and nonnursing). Some applicants don't identify their leadership activities, which can hurt them during scoring of the application.

RISKS AND GUIDELINES

Are clinical nursing instructors "legally bound" to write letters of reference? For the most part, the answer is no. Morally and ethically, though, you need to be willing to write meaningful and relevant reference letters for today's students to help them procure a job. A GPA of 3.99 may look good on a résumé but employers want to know more. How do they function in the real world of acute nursing? How do the patients respond to them as students and caregivers? How do they get along with their peers? Do they exhibit leadership skills on the clinical unit? These strengths (or perhaps weaknesses) cannot be garnered from a GPA.

Nursing is such a unique profession utilizing cognitive and interactional skills that employers are now looking for the total package. Most prospective employers invite each candidate in for an interview where the candidate may face up to six interviewers at one time. Another institution may do group interviews, where each candidate is asked to answer questions in a group setting.

Guidelines to decide if you are in a position to write a letter of reference for a former student would be to pose the following questions to yourself before agreeing to write a letter:

- Do you really know the student well enough to describe his or her abilities in a positive and convincing manner?
- Can you be forthright in your letter and deliver an accurate and positive portrayal of the student?
- Can you meet the student's response time frame for this employer, which often is less than 1 week?

An affirmative answer to each of the above questions usually means that you are an appropriate choice to write this important document.

A WORD TO THE WISE

To save yourself countless tears and "emergency" emails and calls, establish clear, written guidelines for your students for distribution on orientation day. A sample guideline could be:

> I am available to write reference letters after you have completed your clinical rotation with me. I need a minimum of 2 weeks notice, a written request from you stating to whom the letter should be addressed, what position you are applying for, and your signature giving me permission to write the reference letter. (Note: An email request is an appropriate alternative.)

Most employers want to see school letterhead on all letters of reference and many prefer a paper letter. Keep a file of these written requests or a folder on your computer labeled "requests for letters of reference." You may currently be on the best of terms with the student requesting the reference letter, but later on, if the student does not get the desired job, your status may change. Maybe your letter describes quite accurately a moderately successful student. If that student does not get the job, your accurate letter may be fuel for the student's anger. Having the ability to produce a signed request from the student will save you much angst in defending your role in the hiring process. Remember too that phone references absolutely need a signed specific release from the student.

RECOMMENDATIONS REQUESTED BY "NOT-SO-HIGH FLIERS"

Sally, that personable and fun student who gave you that Starbucks gift card as a token of appreciation after her clinical rotation, now asks you to write a reference letter in connection with a job application for the intensive care unit (ICU) of a very busy center-city hospital. As much as you truly enjoyed this student's company, she was not the most competent and skilled practitioner. You could see Sally doing well on a slower-paced community hospital's transitional care unit, but not in the hectic environment of a metropolitan ICU. What do you do? Do you exaggerate or "stretch" the truth about Sally's abilities? Ethically, you can't. Remember that you are being trusted by employers to give an accurate description of your students. Indirectly, but more importantly, you are being trusted by the patients your student will care for. Rather than write a letter that you do not feel comfortable with, why not change gears and engage in some career counseling? You could speak with Sally and communicate your heartfelt belief that she will make a wonderful nurse who will enjoy a long career in the right setting. Although there is no guarantee as to how your response for a letter of recommendation will be received in such an instance, there is no denying that your student will benefit the most from this honest answer.

COMPONENTS OF A GOOD LETTER OF REFERENCE

A good letter of reference will simply tell the truth. If you do not remember the student's performance, say so to the student. Give examples of the student's work when you write your letter. For example, if the student is applying to work on an oncology unit and she cared for a patient with cancer during your clinical, give that experience as an example. If the student assisted all of his peers and the staff in an above average manner, give that as an example. If the student rarely was on time for clinical, you may want to refer to the fact that "early morning" hours may not be the best shift for this student. It usually will be up to the student to decide to submit your letter.

It is best to state in the reference letter that you are writing at the request of (name of student) and include the capacity in which you know the student (e.g., I was her first medical-surgical clinical instructor in her junior year). See Appendix D: Sample Letters of Reference. Be sure to use nursing school letterhead.

Another tip would be to specify what job or position your reference is intended to cover. For example, if writing a letter for a new graduate, state that this student would be a qualified and excellent candidate for a new graduate position at your facility. That will prevent your letter from being misconstrued as a blanket recommendation that would include a more advanced position for a new graduate.

Ideally, you will be writing the letter to a specific person for a specific job. However, that ideal is not always the best fit in meeting student needs. Sometimes students request a more general reference letter when they are applying to multiple facilities at multiple locations. In this situation, be accurate and specify that the letter is written for a new nurse graduate and simply describe your experience with him or her.

Today, many students requesting reference letters must waive their right to read the reference from you. Still, be cautious about what you write and only write exactly what you can support. One never knows what path this letter may take and who may ultimately read it! When no such waiver exists, it is best practice to give the student a copy of your letter before you send it to the employer. That way, if the student does not like what you have written, he or she can choose not to include your reference.

HOW TO POLITELY SAY "NO"

Suppose a student requests that you write a letter of reference for a job. Unfortunately, this student barely passed your clinical. So, how can you write a letter of reference on this student's behalf? Are you required to do so? Unless a given nursing school's policy in this regard says otherwise, the answer is *no*—you are not required to write a letter of reference for any student. To avoid hurt feelings, try a subtle escape. You might say to the student that you do not feel that you are the best person to write the letter of reference, and that a different instructor with whom the student has had a more positive experience may be a better choice. If the student insists that the letter should come from you, you can write one that simply describes the clinical that you taught, that the student "arrived every day and was on time" if in fact that was the case. When that is the extent of your letter, the nurse recruiter will be able to ascertain your unwritten sentiments and, hopefully, the student will too.

GET THAT LETTER INTO THE MAIL

Pay attention to submission timeline requirements. Even a sparkling letter of reference can lose its luster if submitted late. At the same time, tardy reference requests on the part of students and your own conflicting professional priorities can sometimes make late submissions inevitable. In cases where you are simply too swamped to get a letter of reference out on time, follow up as soon as possible and apologetically explain your plight to place the "blame" where it belongs.

Considering the importance that letters of reference play in nursing job prospects, give serious consideration to these requests as you receive them, and do your best to provide an accurate and timely portrayal of your students in any letter that you do choose to write.

FAST FACTS in a NUTSHELL

- Establish guidelines for reference letters on your orientation day with student groups.
- In composing letters of reference, state the truth and give specifics when possible.
- Politely say "NO" to a reference letter request with which you are not comfortable.

20

Role of Simulation

Clinical learning using simulation has risen in popularity. Schools have considered using simulation as a substitute or a possible "make-up" for a clinical day. This chapter will explore the current use of simulation and the overall role it currently has in many nursing programs.

In this chapter, you will learn:

1. The utility of simulation as an instructional method
2. The pros and cons of using simulation to practice patient care
3. The basic application of simulation in clinical education

Simulators and simulation-type experiences are not a new phenomenon to many professionals. Simulations have been present in society for some time, as the airline industry and the military have used simulated environments to prepare their pilots or their military personnel for certain real-life scenarios (Hayden, 2010). In addition, the methods integrated in the "simulated" learning experience, such as role play, have been around since the advent of pedagogy and higher education methods. Role play has long been used by nurse educators as a teaching strategy, in which students take on roles and practice these roles based on various patient cases, or by further developing a scenario that may have occurred during that week's clinical practice experience. However, with enhanced technology, role playing in nursing education has expanded to incorporate a lab setting with manikins and various other equipment. This type of learning has been integrated in many nursing programs as part of the "simulation" experience. To create more realism in these simulated experiences, various acute to more complex patient scenarios have been incorporated, as well as key practice aspects that you may find in many hospital settings. In various nursing textbooks, you will see simulations described as "clinical simulations" or "simulation scenarios."

Simulations are events that provide opportunities for students to think and care for diverse patients in a nonthreatening, safe, and controlled environment (Jeffries, 2005). It can be seen as an instructional method that supplements learning outside of the usual classroom lecture, or as an instructional method that can highlight particularly difficult subject matter such as end-of-life care, care of the acutely ill patient, or culturally sensitive care.

Today, the use of simulation in nursing education has greatly expanded. In the past, simulators were primarily limited to a rubber body or body part such as a model arm or model patient. It then expanded to being more popularly used by various nurse educators who found themselves needing newer ways to teach challenging critical care concepts and to explore real-life patient cases minus the stresses invoked by hospital settings. Simulation labs became commonplace for teaching students critical care concepts (Morton, 1995). Most recently, the use of simulation labs in clinical education is being carefully examined.

A recent survey conducted by one of the authors explored the beliefs and experiences of a clinical group of senior-level student nurses. The survey revealed that many of the group surveyed did not believe a "simulation experience" should ever replace a clinical day. Their comments about the hospital practicum experience were:

- Offers the "reality" aspect not found in simulations
- Nothing can replace the actual experience of working with real people with real issues
- Allows us to see the "big picture" of nursing

These students offered recommendations on the role of simulation without its interference with their clinical practica experience. One viewed simulation as an "adjunct" or a method to practice skills with which they may be having difficulty in the practice setting. Today the literature recognizes that nurse educators are using various types of simulations to supplement their clinical education teaching or as an adjunct to it.

The type of simulation that is selected by the educator depends on the degree of realism (or fidelity) encountered in the event. High-fidelity simulation is the type that has emerged in popularity among nursing programs since the 1990s (Goldsworthy & Graham, 2012), although there are also low- and medium-fidelity simulations. Technology has had a big role in the surge of simulation labs that are commonplace in many prelicensure programs today. In simulation labs, you will find human patient simulators who can talk, have various breath or cardiac sounds, and can perform various other functions. These human patient high-fidelity simulators are attached to cardiac monitors and are operated through computer programs managed by a lab coordinator or someone hired by the school to maintain an adequate simulation environment. They are not seen as the person that leads the simulation for students, but as the lab "coordinator" or "director" who has a primary role in maintaining the appropriate environment and the various equipment.

Although simulation has been welcomed by many nurse educators, there are still challenges faced by nursing programs that wish to use various types of simulations. First and foremost, there must be adequate resources and a designated area specifically designed for these simulation labs. Furthermore, whether low- or high-fidelity simulations are used, someone must be savvy with the various computer-generated programs that are required to run a successful simulation. This person will be employed by the school. He or she must also possess attention to detail in maintaining the various equipment. Last, this person must have the management and communication skills to work with a variety of nursing faculty and students. Certain clinical instructors may be employed in nursing programs where there is a built-in "skills lab" prior to beginning the clinical practicum; it may be the duty of that instructor to visit and orient himself or herself to the simulation lab and to meet any assigned simulation lab personnel.

The prevalence of simulation and its utility in learning environments has been well documented but questions remain regarding the role and outcome of simulation in these environments (Hayden, 2010; Norman, 2012). Many state that the initial simulation experiences were brought on by barriers found in clinical education. There continue to be restrictions imposed by agencies due to the lack of clinical sites that can accommodate students from various nursing programs. Faced with increased enrollment, the faculty shortage, and agency restrictions, clinical simulations are being seen as a teaching and learning strategy. Many are excited about its implications for clinical education and student outcomes, but others are cautious about its overall purpose for knowledge development and thinking in a practice discipline such as nursing.

Educators may say that there are the usual challenges in introducing simulations as people and nurses do not like "change." Let's face it—the traditional ways of teaching are very hard to drop. This instructional method in particular— the traditional clinical education practicum—has been the mainstay for experiential learning and clinical practice for millions of practicing RNs. It is difficult to change the existing mindset. What has been the biggest question is "Can simulated clinical experiences replace the clinical practicum experience?" That is a question that has been debated by professional nurses. There has been no literature that has provided information on the effect of clinical simulation on clinical performance (Norman, 2012). There will hopefully be some preliminary answers soon.

The National Council of State Boards of Nursing (NCSBN) has commissioned a landmark study that will explore critical questions pertaining to simulations. Five associate degree programs and five baccalaureate degree programs were chosen to participate in this national study exploring the role of simulation in prelicensure nursing education. The NCSBN Simulation Study will hopefully give some needed insight to the big questions facing the use of simulation in clinical education and will finally provide some evidence on the comparison of patient care simulations to real-life patient care.

Although the trend in nursing education is to review and understand simulation, without further evidence produced by research studies, nursing programs are, for the most part, using simulation as part of a lab experience for a Health Assessment or Fundamentals course, or as an active learning opportunity to further explore a major concept from didactic instruction. As a result, most state boards have inconsistently addressed simulation use or have no broad regulations identifying implications to clinical education. For example, Ohio specifies that lab hours, not clinical hours, can be used for simulation experiences. In Maryland, schools are not permitted to substitute clinical education hours for simulations.

In New York, simulation is seen as a supplement and not a replacement. According to Boland and Finke (2009), faculty must make difficult decisions about which learning experiences are most influential in developing competent practice nurses.

Hopefully the big questions that apply to clinical education will be addressed by that NCSBN study. Simulations, whether low or high fidelity, are still the main responsibility of full-time teachers and not the adjunct clinical faculty. Until the state boards of nursing provide that language and permit clinical simulations to replace aspects of the clinical education experience, we must continue to teach our students the best way we can. What we can definitely share with our newer clinical faculty hires is the roles of simulations in nursing programs. Share with them that today's students are now practicing assessment and fundamentals skills on a manikin in a simulation exercise during lab hours. Some students who may look relatively comfortable with rapidly changing aspects of their patient care experience may tell you that it is attributed to the simulation lab in the school where full-time teachers were able to assist them to practice with multiple events and patient case scenarios.

Most schools have simulation labs and now many hospitals are also incorporating simulations to reinforce knowledge, advance skills, and evaluate the decision making of their staff personnel. Simulations are here and will not go away. However, it is imperative that all nurse educators in and out of the classroom keep an eye on their learners. The inherent job of the teacher is to know his or her learners and their "level" of learning. Without substantial research evidence and support from the boards of nursing, simulations should not be replacing clinical practicum experiences at this time. Clinical practica provide a colorful array of patient experiences that cannot be fully "simulated" in a lab setting. It has been said that nurses do not practice in a vacuum. Student nurses also should not be in that vacuum.

FAST FACTS in a NUTSHELL

- Simulation provides opportunities to practice nursing skills.
- Using simulations should be based on the level of the learner.
- Clinical instructors should be aware that most students have had simulation experiences as part of their nursing program.

Appendices

A

An Example of Guidelines for Clinical Orientation Day

WELCOME TO 3 C

Orientation day begins at 8 a.m. sharp. Meet at the Barden Lobby. Directions are provided and you also can access the clinical settings website at www.lifecare.org.

September 1, 20XX

This is a regular clinical day with time allocated for lunch. The schedule is 8 a.m. to 2 p.m.

Bring blood pressure cuff, stethoscope, pen, paper, and notebook, and wear full uniform with identification badge per the student handbook.

Expectations for students will be discussed during this orientation day.

Park in the hospital garage; you will receive parking vouchers for each day. They cannot be replaced. The fee for parking is $8.00/day without vouchers.

There will be a medication quiz on this orientation day per level policy. You must pass this quiz to begin giving medications at the site. Safe knowledge and administration of medications are evaluated at all times. You may use a calculator.

3 C is an approximately 30-bed surgical unit. There are also designated beds for short stay after surgical procedures.

Please review surgical procedures in your medical-surgical textbooks. You will probably have an opportunity to irrigate nasogastric tubes, change dressings, provide postop care, give discharge instructions, give subcutaneous insulin and Lovenox, complete assessments, perform sterile gloving for hygiene and personal care, prioritize care, review pain management, go to the operating room and endoscopy unit, and work with a staff nurse.

Please begin to review all of the above procedures. You are expected to review any skill needed in the lab with Marlene if you have any questions or need to practice. I expect you to have reviewed all of the above skills and have practiced in the lab before a clinical opportunity to perform that skill occurs.

This is a fast-paced unit, and there are registered nurses, patient care techs, and aides, and a unit secretary.

Unit coordinator is Diane Marag.

Unit manager is Mary Beth Brouty.

Unit phone number on 3 C is 610-555-36XX.

I look forward to working with you, and the staff on 3 C is happy to be working with you.

Susan Stabler-Haas
Distributed on 8/30/20XX

B

Clinical Journal: NSL/NSG 423

WRITTEN ASSIGNMENT: CLINICAL JOURNAL

Instructor: [Name]

Starting *Week 2* of this rotation: Students must submit a clinical journal on at least one of the clients that they cared for during the previous week. The student must be able to *verbalize* nursing actions and rationale during the clinical day for the patients to whom he or she is assigned. Examples will be provided. Clinical journals are to be submitted weekly on Tuesdays at postconference.

WRITTEN FORMAT OF CLINICAL JOURNAL

Include Your Goals and Objectives for the Week in Your Clinical Journal

1. PATIENT DATA
   a. Diagnoses
   b. PMH/PSH (past medical and surgical history)

   c. Pathophysiology of diagnoses (cite)
   d. Must compare your client's diagnosis to the textbook and cite information from the text (cite source)
2. DOCUMENT "SYSTEMS" ASSESSMENT
   a. (See page 2)

3. DIAGNOSTIC DATA—LABWORK—NURSING IMPLICATIONS
   a. Report *potential* diagnostics pertinent to diagnoses (i.e., chest x-ray results for CHF)
   b. Report any *actual* abnormal lab work and analyze levels r/t client
4. NURSE MANAGEMENT PLAN—Document:
   a. Two priority nursing diagnoses
   b. One STG per each diagnosis (patient outcome) measurable
   c. Two nursing interventions per goal
   d. Evaluate each intervention
5. CLIENT EDUCATION
   a. Identify and analyze teaching needs (actual or potential) of client
6. MEDICATIONS
All medications that the client received during your shift must be listed. You must list the name of the medications, the indication for the medications, lab work needed for this medication, nursing care, and dosage.

Example: Lovenox: Anticoagulant, prevention of thromboembolism phenomena following surgical procedures, prevention of such disorders when patient on bed rest

Labs: Monitor CBC, platelet count, check for black tarry stools, hematuria, fall in blood pressure, signs of bleeding

Nursing: Check for signs of bleeding, gums, stool, urine. Check for bruising

Dosage: SC (adults) 30 mg. Twice daily start within 24 hours of surgery

Antidote: Protamine sulfate

Reason this patient received medication: Patient had surgery and was immobilized, prophylactic.

7. SELF-EVALUATION AND REFLECTION
   (Minimum of two paragraphs)

   Reflect on your week: (a) Pertinent feelings and thoughts about the nursing role. (b) Critique your performance as a student nurse. (c) Did you achieve your goals? (d) What would you do differently? Write as if you were documenting in a log or diary.

   Evaluation Method: Clinical journals will be evaluated based on the evaluative statements from the Clinical Evaluation Tool.

8. EVALUATE the client's psychological health. Ask the two following questions: (a) Have you experienced the feeling of sadness over the last 2 weeks? (b) Have you lost interest in activities or things that you usually enjoy doing?

   Document your assessment of the client's mental state.

C

4 C Clinical Assignment Sheet

Student	Room Number/ Med Assignment	Patient Data
Claire	Day with nurse	Rose or Jan
Kristen	63 **Meds**	This was Claire's patient last week. Resp. failure, post MI, post filter, inf. Vena cava, Isolation (contact), *Clostridium difficile* Meds: Heparin sub-q, heparin IV in PICC line, Protonix IVPB, Lactinex, vancomycin, Vasotec, Lanoxin, Coreg, NovoLog flexpen
Cara	53 54	Pancreatitis, *Clostridium difficile* May have companion with her Did not get diagnosis
Neil	58 **Meds**	Pneumonia, hyponatremia, pulmonary hypertension. Meds: albuterol inhalation, Protonix, Senokot, Solu-Medrol IV (20 mg), Cardizem CD, Colace, Lanoxin, Humibid LA, ASA, Tylenol
Karen	OR	
Amy	59 **Meds**	Recurrent pneumonia, tube feeding via PEG, DSG. Change, Meds: heparin sub-q, heparin IV via PICC, folic acid, Dulcolax supp., Novolin R Innolet, albuterol inhalant, MSO4 IV, lorazepam IV

(*continued*)

Student	Room Number/ Med Assignment	Patient Data	(continued)
Katie	69	Diabetic ketoacidosis, blood sugar of 1100 on 10/30. PICC, MRSA	
Casandra	Endo		
Beth	79 **Meds**	This was Casandra's client last week. Contact isolation. PICC flushed, Nystatin cream, Lopressor, Lasix 40 IVP, Lac-Hydrin 12% topical, alprazolam, albuterol/ipratropium	

D

Sample Letters of Reference

SAMPLE I

September 9, 20XX

To Whom It May Concern:

I am writing this letter of recommendation at the request of Alison Z. It is a pleasure to do so. I know Alison in my capacity as nursing instructor. I taught Alison in her first nursing classroom course, in a summer elective clinical course, and more recently in her first medical-surgical clinical rotation. It is from that perspective that I write this letter.

Alison was a very conscientious and able student in her first nursing course. She provided thorough and well-detailed work and also participated in all student groups. The summer elective clinical course took place at a skilled nursing home and she cared for several totally dependent geriatric clients and provided excellent care. Most recently, I was her clinical instructor at ABC Hospital on an acute surgical floor. She was responsible for two patients on many clinical days, and also administered their medications. She cared for a wide variety of patients and always completed all of her work, providing excellent total nursing care.

The hospital's senior staff nurses complimented her on her willingness to assist all of the staff and for her enthusiasm to learn and provide total care. They encouraged her to submit her résumé to them to be a member of their team. She also submitted excellent journals, which demonstrated a keen ability to correlate textbook knowledge with clinical performance.

Alison is extremely conscientious and well prepared in her interaction with her clients. She is astute and has an above-average ability to understand their medical and nursing needs and deliver outstanding care.

I would strongly recommend Alison for a position as a professional nurse in your facility. If you have any questions, please contact me at 555-525-99XX or my email clinical instructor@university.edu.

Sincerely,

[Instructor name], MSN, RN

SAMPLE 2

March 24, 20XX

To Whom It May Concern:

I am writing this reference letter at the request of Andrea D. It is a pleasure to do so.

I have taught Andie in both the classroom and in the clinical area. She possesses an outstanding ability to thoroughly understand complex subjects and implement this knowledge into the clinical area.

I recently had Andie in her first medical-surgical rotation at ABC Hospital. She was practicing on an acute unit and she had several extremely ill patients. She recently took an elective Critical Care Practicum with me at ABC Hospital. This course was only available to the top tier of our nursing class. It exposed the students to all aspects of critical care nursing. Andie was one of the best students in this rotation and was complimented by the nursing staff.

The primary nurse, a veteran of many years, made a special effort to compliment Andie's abilities and nursing care concerning a particular critical patient.

Andie also has a unique ability to care for the mental and physical components of her patients. It is evident in observing Andie's delivering of patient care that her years of working as an extern have contributed to her excellence.

Andie also is an excellent contributor to all discussions and to classroom interactions. She is articulate and has many leadership qualities.

I would highly recommend Andie to your hospital as a newly graduated professional nurse. If you have any questions, please email me at clinical instructor@university.edu.

Sincerely,

[Instructor name], MSN, RN

References

American Association of Colleges of Nursing. (1999). *AACN position statement. Nursing education's agenda for the 21st century.* Washington, DC: Author.

American Nurses Association. (2001). *Code of ethics for nurses with interpretive statements.* Retrieved March 21, 2008, from http://nursingworld.org/ethics/code/protected_nwcoe813.htm

Boland, D. L., & Finke, L. M. (2009). Curriculum designs. In D. M. Billings & J. A. Halstead (Eds.), *Teaching in nursing: A guide for clinical faculty* (3rd ed., Ch. 8). St. Louis, MO: Saunders Elsevier.

Gaberson, K. B., & Oermann, M. H. (2010). *Clinical teaching strategies in nursing* (3rd ed.). New York: Springer Publishing Company.

Goldsworthy, S., & Graham, L. (2012). *Simulation simplified: A practical handbook for critical care nurse educators.* Philadelphia: Lippincott Williams & Wilkins.

Goleman, D. (1995). *Emotional intelligence.* New York: Bantam Publishing.

Hanna, D. R., & Romana, M. (2007). Debriefing after a crisis. *Nursing Management, 28*(8), 38–42, 44–45, 47.

Hayden, J. (2010). Use of simulation in nursing education: National survey results. *Journal of Nursing Regulation, 1*(3), 52–57.

Ironside, P. M., & McNelis, A. (2009). *Clinical education in prelicensure nursing programs.* New York: National League for Nursing.

Jeffries, P. (2005). A framework for designing, implementing, and evaluating simulations used as teaching strategies in nursing. *Nursing Education Perspectives, 26*(2), 96–103.

Morton, P. (1995). Creating a laboratory that simulates the critical care learning environment. *Critical Care Nurse, 16*(6), 76–81.

Norman, J. (2012). Systematic review of the literature on simulation in nursing education. *ABNF Journal, 23*(2), 24–28.

Oermann, M. H., & Gaberson, K. B. (2013). *Evaluation and teaching in nursing education* (4th ed.). New York: Springer Publishing Company.

Potter, P., Perry, A., Stockert, P., & Hall, A. (2013). *Fundamentals of nursing* (8th ed.). St. Louis, MO: Elsevier.

Scanlon, J. M., Care, W. D., & Gressler, S. (2001). Dealing with the unsafe student in clinical practice. *Nurse Educator, 26*(1), 23–27.

Smith, M. H., McKoy, Y. D., & Richardson, J. (2001). Legal issues related to dismissing students for clinical deficiencies. *Nurse Educator, 26*(1), 33–38.

Teeter, M. (2001). Formula for success: Addressing unsatisfactory clinical performance. *Nurse Educator, 30*(3), 91–92.

Wink, D. M. (1995). The effective clinical conference. *Nursing Outlook, 43*, 29–32.

Index